THE ETHICS
OF GENETIC
ENGINEERING

Other books in the At Issue series:

THE ETHICS
OF GENETIC
ENGINEERING

Lisa Yount, *Book Editor*

Daniel Leone, *President*
Bonnie Szumski, *Publisher*
Scott Barbour, *Managing Editor*

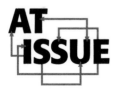

An Opposing Viewpoints® Series

Greenhaven Press, Inc.
San Diego, California

Library of Congress Cataloging-in-Publication Data

The ethics of genetic engineering / Lisa Yount, book editor.
        p. cm. — (At issue)
    Includes bibliographical references and index.
    ISBN 0-7377-0798-4 (pbk. : alk. paper) —
ISBN 0-7377-0799-2 (lib. bdg. : alk. paper)
    1. Genetic engineering—Moral and ethical aspects. I. Yount,
Lisa. II. At issue (San Diego, Calif.)

QH438.7 .E842   2002
174'.966—dc21   2001040466
                                                                             CIP

© 2002 by Greenhaven Press, Inc.
10911 Technology Place, San Diego, CA 92127

Printed in the U.S.A.

Every effort has been made to trace owners of copyrighted material.

Table of Contents

Introduction

In the mid-1970s, the public of the Western world was astonished to learn that scientists had recently invented ways to move pieces of genetic material, the very blueprint of life, from one species to another. Boosters claimed that this new technology of moving and changing genes, which came to be called genetic engineering, would lead to more abundant food supplies, inexpensive medicines, and cures for currently untreatable diseases. Naysayers, on the other hand, feared that it would lead to unstoppable plagues of disease or other environmental disasters.

Supporters and opponents of genetic engineering were just as divided about the basic ethics or morality of the technology as they were about its practical implications. Supporters said it was nothing more than an extension of what breeders of plants and animals had been doing for thousands of years and, indeed, what nature itself did through evolution and natural selection. Detractors claimed that it was "unnatural" and "playing God" and therefore should be banned on ethical as well as safety grounds.

This first wave of concern died down during the 1980s as genetically modified microorganisms were released into the environment and no disasters occurred. Genetic engineers, meanwhile, extended the technology's application from bacteria to plants, mammals, and, ultimately, human cells. Use of transgenic living things—those containing genes from a species other than their own—became a small but growing part of biotechnology, or the use or alteration of other living things in the processes that benefit humankind. For some companies it became very profitable, particularly after the U.S. Supreme Court declared in 1980 that altered living things could legally be patented.

As the twenty-first century begins, genetic engineering has taken over the biotechnology industry so completely that many people now use the terms *genetic engineering* and *biotechnology* interchangeably. Genetically altered crops, including food crops such as soybeans and corn, cover tens of millions of acres in the United States and a few other countries and are marketed around the world. Scientists working for pharmaceutical companies regularly use altered genes to produce "designer" drugs, and other researchers are experimentally treating certain inherited diseases by altering the genes of individuals, a new form of medicine called gene therapy. For better or worse, the next hundred years seem likely to be what longtime genetic engineering foe Jeremy Rifkin calls "the biotech century."

The fact that genetic engineering is so pervasive does not mean that the ethical questions surrounding it have been settled, however. Opponents still question the basic ethics of modifying genes, both because the process creates living things that would never exist in nature and because it threatens to make humans view other life forms or even other human beings as mere manufactured commodities to be changed and discarded at will. Defenders, on the other hand, admit that particular uses of genetic engineering may raise ethical questions but see the process itself as no more unethical than any other form of science or technology. Humans, they say, have always altered their environment to benefit themselves— and genetic engineering, these supporters emphasize, holds the promise of very great benefits indeed, including major new weapons against hunger and disease.

Genetically engineered crops: "Frankenfoods"?

Two particular areas of genetic engineering excite controversy at the dawn of the new century. One is agricultural biotechnology, the production of genetically modified (GM) crops. Criticism has been particularly strong regarding crops used as human food. Protesters in Europe, where many citizens oppose these crops, have dubbed them "Frankenfoods," recalling nineteenth-century English novelist Mary Shelley's prideful scientist and his manufactured monster.

Critics say that creating and growing genetically engineered crops is unethical because the crops threaten the environment. Crops provided with bacterial genes that allow them to make their own pesticides, for example, may result in the death of harmless insects such as monarch butterflies. Genetically engineered food crops, furthermore, may cause unexpected allergic reactions or other harm to human health. These opponents believe that genetically engineered crops should be banned or, at very least, that foods containing GM material should be labeled as such. Supporters of GM crops, however, claim that these threats are unproven or exaggerated and that foods containing GM products do not need to be labeled because they are not different in any important way from their natural counterparts.

A second ethical issue in agricultural biotechnology concerns attempts to encourage poor farmers in developing countries to grow GM crops. Giant corporations such as Monsanto and Novartis own patents on these altered plants. These companies, opponents argue, demand that the farmers buy new seeds each year at premium prices rather than reusing seeds from the previous year's crop as they have traditionally done. The opposition claims that pushing these crops into the developing world will enrich multinational companies at farmers' expense and will not really address the poverty and inequality that are the real roots of world hunger. Biotechnology proponents say that, on the contrary, GM crops offer the world's best chance to end or greatly reduce hunger and malnutrition. They point, for example, to "golden rice," genetically engineered to provide extra vitamin A and therefore prevent a form of blindness, caused by a deficiency of this vitamin, that is widespread among the poor in developing countries.

Altering human genes: "Designer babies"?

Ethical debates perhaps even more bitter than those over GM foods surround the alteration of human genes. Some of these debates are extensions of those that have raged for decades over abortion and reproductive technologies such as in vitro ("test tube") fertilization. Others are as new as human genetic engineering itself.

Alteration of genes in an individual's somatic (body) cells was used successfully to treat disease for the first time in 1990. Changes in the genes of somatic cells are not passed on to a person's offspring. Although many questions remain about the safety and effectiveness of gene therapy, which is still primarily in the experimental stage, this type of human gene alteration raises the fewest ethical issues, especially when it is used to treat or prevent an illness that is life threatening and otherwise incurable.

Some critics, however, see gene therapy, however well intentioned, as the first step down a "slippery slope" that could lead to the revival of eugenics, a pseudoscientific practice popular in the late nineteenth and early twentieth centuries. Supporters of eugenics believed that only people with desirable characteristics (as the dominant groups in society defined "desirable") should be allowed to reproduce. Because of eugenic laws in a number of Western countries and states, including some parts of the United States, thousands of people who were developmentally disabled, mentally ill, convicted of crimes, or otherwise classified as "unfit" were forcibly sterilized. In the late 1930s and early 1940s, Nazi Germany took eugenics to its ultimate extreme by not merely sterilizing but killing those it deemed undesirable, which came to include entire ethnic groups. Because eugenics resulted in such obvious ethical abuses, critics say, anything that might revive it, in whatever form, is ethically dubious.

Even among those who do not question the use of gene alteration to prevent or treat serious illness, some say that in the future, if gene therapy (especially gene therapy administered to a developing fetus before it is born) becomes common, defining "illnesses" appropriate for such treatment may become difficult. Genetic predispositions to conditions such as shortness, obesity, or below-average intelligence, now considered normal inheritable characteristics, may become grounds for gene alteration or abortion. Parents able to afford such treatments, furthermore, may choose to have their normal fetuses' genes modified to increase intelligence, beauty, or other features that they find desirable. Some people feel that gene alteration to prevent a minor handicap or to enhance the condition of a normal offspring would be unethical. Others feel it would be just as ethical as wealthy parents' purchasing first-class schooling or other advantages for their children.

Debate becomes even more severe when the question turns to alteration of germline genes—those in sex cells (eggs and sperm), which are passed on to an individual's offspring. Even many people who find alteration of somatic genes ethically acceptable say that germline genes should never be changed. Doing so could have untoward effects, not merely on an individual, but ultimately on the whole of humanity, perhaps even changing "what it means to be human." Supporters of germline gene therapy, however, are excited about the prospect of human beings controlling their own evolution. Altering germline genes, they say, could eradicate deadly inheritable diseases once and for all and make thrilling improvements in human beings' physical and mental health and powers.

A final ethical issue in human genetic engineering centers on cloning, or creating a new individual that has exactly the same genes as an existing one. Human cloning became a real possibility in 1997, when scientists working at the Roslin Institute in Scotland announced that they had cloned a sheep, which they named Dolly, from the mature cell of an adult ewe. Those who oppose human cloning on ethical grounds say that allowing adults to clone themselves would produce confusion about family relationships and encourage parents to regard cloned offspring as products rather than independent human beings. Supporters of cloning say that it would help infertile couples have children that they could produce in no other way and that clones would be no more "subhuman" than identical twins, which are natural clones of each other.

Ethical as well as practical questions about genetic engineering are sure to become more pressing as the technology continues to spread and develop during the upcoming "biotech century." These questions can be discussed intelligently only if people are willing to educate themselves about the science involved and listen to one another's points of view calmly, without being blinded by emotion or misconceptions. This anthology, At Issue: *The Ethics of Genetic Engineering,* provides a variety of viewpoints about the most controversial ethical aspects of this hotly debated technology.

1

Genetic Engineering Can Be Ethical

Fred Edwords

Fred Edwords is the editor of the Humanist, *for which he writes frequently. This article is based on lectures he gave at the National Conference of the American Humanist Association in San Diego, California, in 1998 and at the International Humanist and Ethical Union World Congress in Mumbai, India, in 1999.*

Technology changes ways of living, values, and even religion. The numerous advances in biotechnology and genetic engineering that have recently taken place or are expected in the near future, such as the mapping of the human genome and genetic modification of plants and animals, are bound to bring many such changes. They raise important ethical issues, including the question of whether living things, even human children, will come to be regarded as mere products. While this new technology should be embraced, it should be shaped thoughtfully by an informed public.

To most people, it doesn't make much sense to compare religion and technology. Each seems to pertain to its own separate sphere. And whenever a connection is noticed, it usually amounts to a recognition that religion uses technology to more effectively propagate its ideas.

Few will deny, however—when pondering these two separately—that each has shown itself capable of affecting the way people think and act. Religion, by its very nature, is intent on the inculcation of specific systems of belief and behavior. But technology—while rarely created with conscious philosophical, psychological, or sociological aims—manages nonetheless to critically impact these areas. A glance at a few recent technological developments and the revolution in values and life-styles each has generated will suffice to make the point.

Technology changes ways of thinking

In the early 1960s, the birth control pill became widely available. This brought increased attention to and acceptance of contraception and fam-

From "How Biotechnology Is Transforming What We Believe and How We Live," by Fred Edwords, *The Humanist*, September 1999. Reprinted by permission of the author.

ily planning, giving women more control over their bodies. It also reduced the risk of pregnancy for those wishing to enjoy sex outside marriage. Soon afterward, we saw family size in the developed nations shrink, sexual freedom expand, and the women's rights movement rise to social prominence. Today, all over the world, values about sex, the family, population growth control, and gender roles are changing or are already dramatically different from what they were prior to that tumultuous decade.

Subsequent to the introduction of the pill, there have been other reproductive technologies: safer abortion procedures, ultrasonography, amniocentesis [a technique that allows detection of some inborn defects before birth], sperm and egg banks, in vitro fertilization, surrogate parenting, fertility drugs, and, soon, advance selection of the gender of one's offspring. Such developments continue to force a host of additional moral and legal issues upon us—requiring further changes or modifications in our ethical standards, social norms, and laws.

The majority of us will think and live very differently tomorrow because of the technologies assimilated into our culture today.

Looking at the broader category of medical technology, we can see that an even greater number of unanticipated moral dilemmas have come up—some of which affect areas so foundational that professionals can disagree on when a person comes into existence and when a person actually dies. Does "human personhood" begin at conception, at the appearance of brain waves, at birth, or possibly at some time after? What we conclude affects our views concerning the freezing of embryos, the rights of such embryos, fetal adoption, a mother's prenatal care obligation, abortion, the atmosphere in the birthing room, and selective nontreatment of severely disabled newborns. Does human life end with the death of the heart, the death of the brain, or the loss of "significant life"? What we determine affects our views on hospice, living wills, withdrawal of life support, suicide, and physician-assisted dying. Soon it may even force us to decide whether or not it is acceptable to use comatose individuals as "living" organ banks.

On a different front, global satellite communication has made the world smaller and has increased public awareness of certain international developments. We can now watch a war or a democratic revolution as it happens, and from both sides. And we can see more directly how actions taken in one place affect the environment or politics in another. This can't help but to advance globalism.

Through the video cassette recorder and cable and satellite television, individual choice in information gathering has been enhanced. As a consequence, people find it easier to get their ethics, aesthetics, and politics from something other than the usual common sources. And in so doing, they come to have a greater vested interest in the preservation of individual liberty, freedom of choice, and minority rights.

Computers expand the range of choice even further. The Internet makes individual information gathering, communication, and idea sharing much easier, even bringing the world to one's home or office. And through desktop publishing or the establishment of a presence on the World Wide Web, any computer owner can become an idea or information disseminator. Virtual communities on the Internet give further support to meeting the needs and upholding the rights of minorities.

Meanwhile, space travel, which has provided humanity with a consciousness-raising view of the Earth from the moon, will eventually do much more. Our species won't be limited only to this planet for its pursuits and interests. Colonies in space will—as have distant colonies throughout human history—bring into existence alternative societies and novel ideas, causing different visions of life's purpose to emerge and be shared.

Clearly, then, technology changes society and values. And it often does so in ways that confront old beliefs head on, bringing about significant societal anxiety. As Alvin Toffler explains in his 1980 best seller *The Third Wave:*

> It is precisely the collapse of the industrial era mind-structure, its growing irrelevance in the face of new technological, social, and political realities, that gives rise to today's facile search for old answers, and to the continual stream of pseudo-intellectual fads that pop up, flash, and consume themselves at high speed.

These, he argued, are the death spasms of an old order in the process of being supplanted by a new.

A few people in the future, as always, will stand by their traditional verities and life-styles, entrenched in their special ways of living in their separate communities, much as the Amish do today. But the majority of us will think and live very differently tomorrow because of the technologies assimilated into our culture today. As Toffler says, "Powerful forces are streaming together to alter social character, to elicit certain traits, to suppress others, and in the process to transform us all."

Among the transformed will be institutions such as the church, which, in order to survive, will eventually need to accommodate these changes (its divines likely proclaiming that the new ideas had really been those of the church all along). Indeed, the necessary debates among the faithful are already in progress.

Technology, then—along with the scientific discoveries that make it possible—not only affects the way people think and act, as religion does, but often forces religion itself to evolve. Back in 1877, Robert Ingersoll put it this way:

> Where once burned and blazed the bivouac fires of the army of progress, now glow the altars of the church. The religionists of our time are occupying about the same ground occupied by heretics and infidels of one hundred years ago. The church has advanced in spite, as it were, of itself. It has followed the army of progress protesting and denouncing, and had to keep within protesting and denouncing distance.

Today's technology also works rapidly. While at one time a vigorous new religion could transfigure a continent in a few centuries, a vigorous new technology can now do the same to the entire world in a matter of decades. Specifically, it took hundreds of years for ideas attributed to a man called Jesus (and others in his camp) to change the face of Europe. But the entire globe was altered in a mere twenty years by the technological innovations of a man named Bill Gates (and others in his field).

The biotechnology revolution

Now, as we enter the twenty-first century, it is becoming clear that the next scientific development ready to metamorphose our ideas and lives is biotechnology. A simple review of developments already in place will make this plain.

As the history of the biotech revolution is now tracked, it is generally said to have gotten underway in 1971 when Ananda Chakrabarty, a microbiologist from India, applied for a U.S. patent on a microorganism he had genetically engineered to eat ocean oil spills. When the patent office rejected his application on the grounds that living things aren't patentable, Chakrabarty appealed. In a close decision, the Court of Customs and Patent Appeals supported his patent request, declaring that, although his microorganism has life, this is "without legal significance" because Chakrabarty's invention is "more akin to inanimate chemical compositions such as reactants, reagents, and catalysts, than to horses and honeybees or raspberries and roses."

In response, the patent office appealed, and the case was eventually heard by the U.S. Supreme Court. In its five-to-four decision in 1980, the High Court granted the patent, arguing that "the relevant distinction was not between living and inanimate things" but whether a "human-made invention" was or wasn't involved. This ruling provided the legal groundwork for all life-form patents since.

And it set off a business frenzy. Later that year Genentech, a genetic engineering firm without a single product on the market, went public, selling shares on Wall Street for $35 apiece. The value rose to $89 per share in the first twenty minutes of trading and Genentech ended the day $36 million richer.

The gene that produces light in the firefly was inserted into the genetic code of a tobacco plant, resulting in tobacco leaves that glow in the dark.

Seven years later, the U.S. patent office issued a ruling that even animals are potentially patentable. A year after that, in 1988, the first mammal was patented: the "onco-mouse," genetically engineered with human genes to predispose it to developing cancer. It is sold as a research model for use in cancer studies. This was soon followed by "AIDS mouse," a research animal that expresses the virus [that causes AIDS] in every cell of its body and passes the virus on to subsequent generations. As Jeremy Rifkin notes in his 1998 book *The Biotech Century*, "Nearly two hundred genetically modified animals, including pigs, cows, and sheep, are awaiting patent approval in the U.S."

But let's go back a step. Chakrabarty's oil-eating microorganism is a relatively simple affair. The real scientific breakthrough occurred in 1973 when biologists Stanley Cohen and Herbert Boyer stitched together pieces of DNA from two unrelated organisms. This launched the field of recombinant DNA surgery, also know as gene splicing. So far, this process is the most dramatic instrument in the growing biotech toolbox.

With these developments came an explosion of activity, the most dramatic of which was the creation of trans-species hybrids—two unrelated life forms genetically blended into chimeras, original species that can't breed or evolve naturally. In 1983, "super mice" were developed by Ralph Brinster of the University of Pennsylvania Veterinary School by inserting human growth hormone genes into mouse embryos. This whole new species of mouse grows twice as fast and almost twice as large as other mice, and the human growth hormone is passed naturally to its offspring. Generations have now come and gone and this unique animal is still thriving.

While some people wish they were never born, an awful lot of people want never to die.

Early in 1984, British scientists fused embryo cells from a sheep and a goat, then implanted the novel embryo into a surrogate animal. A chimeric sheep-goat was born. And later, in 1986, the ultimate trans-species hybrid was created: a life form made from an animal and a plant. Believe it or not, the gene that produces light in the firefly was inserted into the genetic code of a tobacco plant, resulting in tobacco leaves that glow in the dark!

Another significant development was the first government-approved release into the open environment of a genetically engineered organism. This occurred in 1983 with the test release of a bacterium that, when sprayed on crops, prevents frost damage. The mining industry at this time also entered the biotech era. While extracting ores from rock has been a difficult task—involving miners, machines, and long periods of toil—that approach may be coming to an end. Tests have been conducted with bacteria that produce enzymes that eat away the impurities in certain low-grade ores, leaving the pure ore behind. This "bioleaching" could provide a cheap way to extract and process precious metals.

A medicine-related biotechnological development was that of xeno-transplants—the transplanting of organs from one species into another. This came to the public's attention in 1984 with the case of Baby Faye, a fifteen-day-old infant who received a baboon heart to replace her own. Though she died twenty days later, a thirty-five-year-old man received a baboon liver in 1992 and lived for two and a half months. The goal of all this is to create a large supply of genetically modified animal organs that won't be rejected by the human body, thus reducing the wait for and expense of human organs in transplant surgery.

On the international political scene, the biological arms race can be said to have come into its own in the fall of 1984. Secretary of Defense Caspar Weinberger reported to Congress "new evidence that the Soviet Union has maintained its offensive biological warfare programs and that it is exploring genetic engineering to expand its program's scope." In response, the United States launched an effort to close the "gene gap," greatly expanding the Pentagon's budget for "defensive" biological warfare research. In 1981 that budget had been a mere $15.1 million; by 1986 it was up to $90 million. And in that year, the U.S. Department of Defense issued a report stating that genetic engineering, particularly recombinant DNA gene splicing, was making biological warfare practical. Not only were genetic engineers cloning massive quantities of "traditional" pathogens but they were inventing new "designer agents." Just as "designer drugs" were on the market, so were these new biowarfare weapons. They could be created quickly and cheaply, yet antidotes to each might take decades to develop.

In 1995, the Central Intelligence Agency reported its suspicions that seventeen countries besides the United States—Bulgaria, China, Cuba, Egypt, India, Iran, Iraq, Israel, Laos, Libya, North Korea, Russia, South Africa, South Korea, Syria, Taiwan, and Vietnam—were researching or stockpiling germ warfare weapons. More recently, a February 1998 report in the *Baltimore Sun* discusses the April 2, 1979, accidental release of anthrax from a Soviet laboratory in Sverdlovsk, Russia. The significant issue in this incident is that the airborne anthrax germs in question may have been specifically bred by the Soviet military to be resistant to antibiotics and specially engineered to attack adult males. Antibiotics failed to prevent the deaths of over 1,000 civilians, but three times as many men died as women and not a single child fatality occurred.

Changing human genes

After the watershed innovations of the 1970s and 1980s, a plethora of new applications and secondary developments followed immediately. For example, the U.S. Human Genome Project, an effort to spell out the entire genetic code of *Homo sapiens,* began its first phase in 1990. Though the project initially progressed slowly, with a projected completion date of 2005, biologist Craig Venter began in 1991 to use a new process of his own that dramatically accelerated results. As a consequence, newly discovered human gene sequences are being posted on the Internet daily. [The U.S. government and Celera Genomics, Venter's private company, jointly declared the Human Genome Project as completed in June 2000.]

Looking ahead, philosopher of science Philip Kitcher has noted how health insurance companies will want to be able to set insurance rates—or deny insurance altogether—based on what genetic predispositions are discovered in the genetic codes of individual people. And this level of unacceptable discrimination, he optimistically suggests, could force a national health insurance plan to come into existence in the United States.

Meanwhile, Venter has been mapping other organisms. In May 1995 he surprised the scientific world with news that he had deciphered the first complete script of a living organism: the genome of the human pathogen *Haemophilus influenzae.* Since then, his lab has gone on to map the complete genomes of a number of other organisms. He projects that, within the first decade of the twenty-first century, we will know fifty to 100 genomes in nature.

In May 1992 Baby Cloe was born in London. Cystic fibrosis [a severe

inherited disease] ran in the family but the use of abortion for genetic selection had been bypassed through the use of pre-implantation genetic
testing. That is, several eggs had been removed from the mother's womb
and fertilized in vitro with her husband's sperm. The fertilized eggs were
then allowed to develop through the eighth cell division. After that, they
were tested for cystic fibrosis. Two of the embryos were without the disease so they were implanted in the mother. One developed and was born.
Today pre-implantation genetic screening is used regarding a number of
genetic diseases, including sickle-cell anemia and Tay-Sachs.

---

*People will cease to place a premium value on their
"natural" attributes over those which have been
acquired synthetically.*

Besides this neo-eugenic approach to genetic diseases, biotech cures
that don't affect heredity have also been developed. One is the genetic
engineering of a human growth hormone. Originally intended to help
the thousands of U.S. children born with dwarfism, it was patented in the
1980s. By the end of the 1990s, however, its wider use among nonaffected
children resulted in $500 million in sales.

And this introduces an ethical concern. Family doctors and pediatri-
cians are increasingly designating children as abnormal who fall in the
bottom 3 percent of the height scale for their age group. This common
shortness, being defined now as an "illness," results in the growth hormone being more frequently prescribed. It also results in a change in our
notions of "normal." Robin Marantz Henig, writing in the May 1998 *Discover* magazine, notes that this is "a common theme in medical history"—
a treatment developed to resolve an abnormality is eventually used to enhance or standardize normality.

It was, in fact, this very question that induced the National Institutes
of Health to bring researchers and ethicists together in September 1997
for the first Gene Therapy Policy Conference. This was followed two
weeks later by an American Association for the Advancement of Science–
sponsored colloquium on gene alterations directed at the eggs, sperm,
and zygotes [fertilized eggs]—interventions that could, if developed,
change an individual's heredity and hence the genetic endowment of future generations. Many speakers at these gatherings expressed concern
that the use of such technology could result in a "biological reinforcement" of socioeconomic and class distinctions. After all, gene therapy
would most often benefit those most able to pay for it. Furthermore,
people seem to desire such choices. As Henig reports:

> More than 40 percent of Americans, according to a March of
> Dimes survey, think it would be okay to use gene therapy to
> make their children either more attractive or more intelligent
> than they were otherwise destined to be. A Gallup poll of
> British parents found many of them also willing to consider
> such genetic "enhancement," and for some surprising and
> rather disconcerting reasons: 18 percent to change a child's

aggression level or remove a predisposition to alcoholism, 10 percent to keep a child from becoming homosexual, and 5 percent to make a child more physically attractive.

As if to show how close such developments might be to reality, researchers at Case Western Reserve University Medical School in Cleveland, Ohio, in April 1997 created the first artificial human chromosome. This could eventually be instrumental in the customized design of genetic traits in embryos or even in sex cells before conception. Artificial chromosomes could then become genetic "cassettes" that would alter people's genetic inheritance, wiping out genetic diseases in family lines but also doing many other things.

Some suggest that this could have negative fallout regarding society's tolerance for disability. To see this, we need only look back at the year 1975, when Paul and Shirley Berman sued two New Jersey doctors for "wrongful life." The Bermans argued that their daughter, who was born with Down's syndrome, would have been aborted had their doctors advised the amniocentesis that would have detected the condition. They thus charged that the doctors had been negligent and had contributed to a "wrongful birth." Although the Bermans lost the substance of their suit, the New Jersey Supreme Court did award them "emotional damages" for their suffering. Since then, many states have recognized a child's right to bring "wrongful life" lawsuits on his or her own behalf.

A series of problems

Of course, while some people wish they were never born, an awful lot of people want never to die. That's why the announcement by scientists in California and Texas in March 1998 is so interesting. Through direct genetic manipulation of a human DNA molecule, these molecular biologists were able to extend cell growth and postpone cell death to a point nearly twice what is normal. With further research and development, this process could allow humans to almost double their lifespans—raising a host of cultural, economic, ethical, political, and religious problems. Not the least of these would be the need to dramatically slow the birthrate. On a more mundane level, retirement plans and the Social Security system would have to be overhauled. (And with copyrights now extending to the lifetime of the author plus seventy years, this article might not enter the public domain until around 2150!)

If such neo-eugenic and Fountain of Youth issues still have a ring of science fiction to them, this cannot be said for the entrenched place biotechnology has already established for itself in medicine. In 1995, over 280 new genetically engineered medicines were tested—a 20 percent increase over the previous year. Now millions of people use gene-spliced drugs and medications to treat AIDS, cancer, heart disease, kidney disease, strokes, and the like. The new medicines have, in some cases, replaced the old. For instance, genetically engineered human insulin, used in treating diabetes, has all but replaced that derived directly from animals.

In May 1997, U.S. scientists isolated a gene that regulates muscle growth in mice. It was then learned that, with this gene removed, mice can grow stronger and develop bulging muscles, huge shoulders, and broad hips. The new breed of muscular rodent was dubbed "Mighty Mouse" and will soon be used to develop new treatments for muscle-related diseases such as muscular dystrophy. (Of course, as soon as it is used for that, someone will develop an application to enhance the performance of healthy athletes.)

More than ever before, we will be able to evolve whatever we want—or simply manufacture it directly.

In 1999 at the Tufts School of Veterinary Medicine in Massachusetts, pigs genetically altered with human genes were being bred in the hope of producing a universal organ donor for human beings—a donor that can be raised in large supply on special farms. This could also increase the supply and lower the cost of transplant organs. Of course, cross-species organ donation brings with it the risk of cross-species infection. This is why the U.S. Food and Drug Administration (FDA) has been drawing up guidelines.

On a parallel track is the creation of new bio-synthetics. Artificial skin is a prime example. Cultured and grown in laboratories, it is now used to treat burn victims. In 1996 a patient with severe burns over 60 percent of his body was treated in San Diego, California, with artificial skin. He was able to be released from the hospital only forty-seven days later.

The goal of those developing this latter technology is to make organs rather than transplant them. Research is now underway to fabricate heart valves, ears, noses, breasts, wombs, and other body parts. Robert Pool, in the May 1998 *Discover*, notes that Joseph Vacanti, chief of organ transplantation at Children's Hospital in Boston and a developer of synthetic organs, believes that someday "we will have cell banks with cells that have been genetically engineered to be invisible to the human immune system. To create a liver or kidney or heart, a tissue engineer would withdraw correct cells from the cell bank, seed them into an organ framework, and grow the organ."

But again, what starts out as a solution to a disability appearing at birth, during maturation, or after injury is quickly enlisted in the service of those able-bodied individuals who desire some healthful improvement or cosmetic enhancement. And to the extent that such technology becomes relatively cheap and widely available, people will cease to place a premium value on their "natural" attributes over those which have been acquired synthetically. Consider fashion modeling. Many still discuss whether this or that individual is "real" or "plastic." Over time, however, it's quite possible that such a distinction will cease to have any interest or even meaning.

Living things—or products?

Besides affecting what we are, biotechnology is affecting what we eat—so much so that in 1992, when the FDA announced that it wouldn't require the special labeling of genetically modified (GM) foods, there was an outcry from critics concerned about the possible transfer of allergens [substances that can cause allergic reactions] through the gene-splicing process. A 1996 study then proceeded to confirm that this had, in fact, already happened. So the FDA altered its position, requiring the labeling of all GM foods that use the genetic code of known allergenic organisms.

Since then the FDA has approved numerous GM crops for sale in the United States—and they're being used. GM corn was grown in 1997 on over 3.5 million acres and soy on more than eight million acres. The majority of U.S. farmland could be converted to this type of agriculture in less than five years.

Such development, however, has caused opposition in Europe and Asia. For example, in early 1999, a number of large European grocery chains vowed to go "GM free," making long-term contracts with growers to provide GM-free produce. Meanwhile, in India, as activists set fire to suspected fields of GM crops, the Indian Supreme Court upheld a ban on GM crop testing. Under all this pressure, a number of large multinational corporations—including Cadbury-Schweppes, Gerber, Nestle, and Unilever—have suddenly joined the GM-free consortium. The social controversy over "Frankenfood" is well underway.

Besides enhancing food quality and crop yields, another important aspect of agricultural biotechnology is the creation of pest- and virus-resistant—as well as herbicide-tolerant—plants. But natural plant plasticity poses a special danger here. Pollen from crops engineered to be resistant to weed killer have been known to fertilize related weeds, creating superweed hybrids that are also resistant to weed killer.

With the capacity to massively change the external world of animals and plants to suit our desires, we relinquish another level of our ties to the land and external nature.

Crops are also being aided by the use of special defensive strategies against insects. A predator mite was the first genetically engineered insect to be released. It was let loose in Florida in 1996 in the hope it would eat other mites that damage crops. In California, a lethal gene has been inserted into the crop-damaging pink bollworm. The genetically altered caterpillars, when released into the general population, become moths and then mate. The resulting offspring are expected to experience a massive die-off, allowing cotton crops to grow in an environment more benign. Meanwhile, scientists continue to work on the creation of harmless disease-bearing insects.

Down on the farm these days, not only are the plants more productive but so are the animals. Australian scientists have engineered a breed of pigs that is 30 percent more efficient and can be brought to market seven weeks earlier than ordinary pigs. They have also made sheep that grow 30 percent faster and will soon make their wool grow faster as well. In the United States, a new breed of turkey hen has been created that lays more eggs because it no longer engages in "non-productive" mothering activity over them.

Besides being designed in the laboratory, useful plants and animals continue, as always, to be discovered or rediscovered in nature, the critical genes being extracted for various purposes. Toward this end, over 400,000 seeds from all over the world have been collected in the U.S. National Seed Storage Laboratory. This is literally a gene bank—as are many others the world over, some of which store rare microorganisms and animal embryos. In related work, there is the Human Genome Diversity Project—an effort to secure blood samples from the world's 5,000 linguistically distinct human populations in the hopes of isolating desirable genes that can be useful in future designer gene projects, especially in medicine.

Pharmaceutical farming

Also for medical purposes, nonhuman animals are being used as living laboratories. This is called pharmaceutical farming or pharming. Whole herds and flocks can produce medicines and nutrients. For example, in April 1996 Grace was born, a transgenic goat with a gene that produces an anti-cancer drug now being tested. Then in February 1997 Rosie was born, a transgenic calf that produces milk containing the necessary nutrients for premature infants who cannot nurse. By 1999, transgenic pigs could produce human hemoglobin.

In order to be effective and guarantee quality control, pharming will require cloning the new ideal animal once it is perfected. That's where the February 1997 birth of Dolly comes in. Dolly was reported as the first cloned mammal, a sheep. Shortly after Dolly came Polly, a cloned sheep that features a customized human gene in its biological code. Then in January 1998 came Charlie, George, and Albert, three cloned calves produced at Advanced Cell Technology, a Massachusetts biotech firm. In 1998 and 1999, goats and mice were cloned. The National Institutes of Health has funded two projects to clone rhesus monkeys. The result of all this is that we will soon mass produce customized animals for a variety of purposes.

Such large-scale creation, use, and manipulation of the flora and fauna of Earth cannot help but have a profound effect on the way we regard all life forms not ourselves. More than ever before, we will be able to evolve whatever we want—or simply manufacture it directly. This is where we will see the most immediate and profound sociological, psychological, and ethical effects of cloning and other biotechnological developments.

Human cloning isn't likely to be the next big issue, then; such a clone, if fully developed, will probably be seen as an identical twin born later—a view unlikely to have much immediate impact on basic human rights. But the animal rights movement is in a wholly different situation. As nonhuman animals come to be regarded as mere bundles of genetic information to be switched, traded, and modified at will—the results therefrom being mass produced and harvested—they will lose much of their status as distinct species, each with a special integrity worth preserving and protecting. This will effectively "desacralize" animals in ways that will influence how people in the future will view them.

The environmental movement will also be affected by this as talk turns from preserving nature in some past "pristine" state to consciously creating exactly the sort of "nature" we want. Debate over the relative merits of preservation ecology, restoration ecology, and inventionist ecology will then become part of common public discourse.

As should be obvious at this point, it isn't farfetched to predict a host of transformations in the way we live and think emerging out of biotechnology. We are already at a time when parents have more and more control over the genetic makeup of their children, designer animals are being created for a variety of technological purposes, designer foods and medicines are being engineered for our physical and mental health, and synthetic human tissues are being developed for restorative as well as cosmetic purposes. We also face new forms of biological pollution, newly engineered pests, and the growing dangers of biochemical war and terrorism. Perhaps sooner than we expect, genetic screening will accompany intelligence testing. And biochemical (or nanotechnological) computers and toys may replace some of those now made of metal and plastic.

Regarding this latter prediction, the handwriting is clearly on the wall. In 1994, Dr. Leonard Adelman at the University of Southern California got a strain of DNA to solve a simple mathematical puzzle. Shortly thereafter, Richard Lipton at Princeton got DNA to perform more complex functions.

But before molecular and "meat" machines dominate the market, there will still be plenty made of plastic, even if petroleum were to become scarce. Chris Sommerville at the Carnegie Institution of Washington, D.C., saw to that in 1993 when he invented a special type of vegetation. Inserting a plastic-making gene into a mustard plant, he converted it into a living plastics factory. Monsanto hopes to have it on the market by 2003. Meanwhile, ICI, a British firm, has engineered bacteria that can produce biodegradable plastics with varying degrees of elasticity and other characteristics.

A philosophical crisis

Overall, we are becoming the remanufacturers of life and materials on Earth and, in time, will be able to spread our "New Genesis" to Venus and Mars, changing the atmosphere on those planets and terraforming the landscape to suit our own desires.

But this shows that even humanists may face a philosophical crisis in the next century.

In the past, people found meaning in nature by observing its cycles: the changes in seasons and the changing requirements that came with them. People found meaning in human life by meeting the needs of family and community. Later, humanist thinkers came to the conclusion that an increased understanding of human nature could provide an important basis for human values. By learning who we are and how we evolved, it would be possible to get a better idea of what is good for us and what we can reasonably expect from ourselves.

But now, with the capacity to massively change the external world of animals and plants to suit our desires, we relinquish another level of our ties to the land and external nature. With the capacity to reshape ourselves, our family genetic heritage, and our communities, we divorce ourselves from many of the familial duties and social connections that once formed the basis of our behavior. And with the capacity to determine the course of our evolution—not to mention the evolution of other species—we potentially lose some of the evolutionary rationale we may have had for our ethics.

Relevant to this latter point is Edward O. Wilson's 1998 book *Consilience,* in which he argues for an empirical basis for ethics. Within our biology, Wilson sees a human nature that will provide a general basis to work from. This isn't any sort of absolute ethical truth, of course, but it is something a little more solid than social relativism or the shifting sands of consequential and situational ethics. This is also where he develops his view of the genetic basis for those ethical inclinations that Adam Smith termed moral sentiments.

We have, however, been creatively interacting with human nature throughout our prehistory and history by the various selective ways that different cultures have bred, have practiced genocide on other cultures, and the like. How much this process has already modified our nature would be interesting to measure. In any case, it is clear that we have never shied away from exercising our influence—to whatever degree possible—on our genetic heritage, on our growth and development, and on our external environment. As a result, our ethical inclinations—rather than belonging exclusively to some relatively fixed system dating from the Old Stone Age—may be a partially ongoing product of our evolving values since humankind first emerged in Africa.

Whatever the case, with the biotech revolution we find ourselves in the ironic situation of becoming empowered to alter our genetics—and eventually these ethical inclinations—more swiftly and more dramatically than ever before, acquiring this power just as we are beginning to understand the genetic roots and original survival advantages of those same ethical inclinations. Thus we gain a capability to change that which we don't yet fully understand and run the risk of doing what we have mistakenly done in the past: upset the balance of nature, suffer the consequences, then scramble to fix our errors.

In this regard, we might well ask: will we go about this in the ways common to us, letting those people with the most power and money or those who control religious belief decide for all of us?

Clearly, the challenge of tomorrow is a momentous one. It is also an adventure into the unknown. We can embrace this adventure or fear it. Chances are, however, the future will belong to those who embrace it. For it is the embracers who most easily become the shapers.

Perhaps for this reason *Humanist Manifesto II* sets forth an optimistic view of technology, declaring:

> Using technology wisely, we can control our environment, conquer poverty, markedly reduce disease, extend our lifespan, significantly modify our behavior, alter the course of human evolution and cultural development, unlock vast new powers, and provide humankind with unparalleled opportunity for achieving an abundant and meaningful life.

But it still follows with a warning:

> The future is, however, filled with dangers. In learning to apply the scientific method to nature and life, we have

opened the door to ecological damage, overpopulation, dehumanizing institutions, totalitarian repression, and nuclear and biochemical disaster.

The matter warrants our concern and involvement. But if our involvement is to be productive, it needs to be informed. That requires keeping up to date on the revolutions in science and technology that surround us, particularly those in the field of biology. It means looking past the hype—whether of the "gee whiz" or the alarmist variety. It means following the money trail to see where reside the concentrations of power that determine what technologies are used, how they are used, who benefits, and who loses. And it means recognizing that all these factors will directly affect ourselves and our progeny.

For they are doing so already.

2

Genetic Engineering
Is Not Ethical

Martin Teitel, interviewed by Casey Walker

Martin Teitel is executive director of the Council for Responsible Genetics, which works to increase public participation in decisions about genetic engineering and biotechnology. He also edits Genewatch, *an activist journal on biotechnology. His books include* Genetically Engineered Food: Changing the Nature of Nature *(with Kimberly A. Wilson). Casey Walker is editor of* Wild Duck Review, *a magazine that includes essays, memoirs, interviews, and other features providing "wild" thought on contemporary issues.*

The modern worship of technology and progress combine with an outpouring of corporate greed to place the biotechnology revolution on shaky ethical ground. Bioethicists often fail to mention its chief danger, which is the changing of other living things and even human beings into mere commodities. Biotechnology can result in invading people's bodies without consent, as when information about people's DNA is stored in databanks; determining who will be insured, hired, or even born; or even changing the inherited genes that determine the nature of human beings. Living things should be seen in terms of intrinsic worth, not mere usefulness.

Casey Walker: Within our lifetime we've witnessed industry shift its base of power from resource extraction to communications/information, and, recently, to genetic information. Each evolution has been publicly sanctioned by assumptions of inevitability and progress toward a better world. Will you begin by critiquing those same assumptions for biotechnology?

Martin Teitel: The idea of progress is a myth, particularly when you apply it to biology. Human beings construct and reconstruct the world according to their own ideas and cultures and agendas, but the biological world works very differently from the world of human ideas. It operates under a different set of assumptions and principles, which is why the term *genetic engineering* is appropriate. We are teleological [concerned with the ends or purposes of actions]. We march toward goals that we've

From "Framing Ethical Debates," an interview of Martin Teitel by Casey Walker, in *Made Not Born: The Troubling World of Biotechnology*, edited by Casey Walker (San Francisco: Sierra Club Books, 2000). Copyright © 2000 by Wild Duck Review. Reprinted with permission.

decided upon in our minds, and we try to shape and fashion the world to reach those goals. And that's called progress. Putting nature's system of biological processes into an engineering-oriented, teleological-oriented, and progress-oriented framework is, I think, destructive by definition. It's degenerative. I'm not making out some kind of romantic, Rousseauistic case that we should all wear animal skins and run around in the forest. I have my laptop computer and my Dodge van. But there's a big difference between living in and learning from the world, and shaping that world so that it "lives" within our ideas, which is precisely what genetic engineering does.

David Noble's books World Without Women *and* The Religion of Technology *trace historical shifts in religious and political power from the embodied world to the technological world—assumptions so deeply ingrained and part of our milieu that we rarely question them. How do you see the critique of biogenetic engineering becoming proactive along these lines?*

One of the reasons I like to talk about slippery slopes is that we have been sliding on a slippery slope for a long time: the upper end of our slippery slope is the adoption of science as a religion and the consequent impoverishment of our epistemology [study of the sources, nature, and limits of knowledge]. At the root of this process, our ways of knowing have become constrained. Those who go outside the approved epistemology are labeled as heretical and are treated the way heretics have been treated for thousands of years, whether it's through the denial of tenure, or the kind of frothing, hysterical editorial about Jeremy Rifkin (author of *The Biotech Century*) that appears in the *Wall Street Journal* from time to time. I call it religion because, ironically, it's based on faith more than on assumptions. This is okay for people to do, I suppose, but it may be the first religion in history with a core built upon the denial it's a religion.

When we have the coupling of a shaky social and values mechanism with a fierce engine of acquisition and possession, we get something very ugly.

And criticism of it is dismissed as "retro," as Luddite, rather than genuinely turning our attention to the ethical and intellectual debates essential to the world we are creating.

Yes. There are really two things operating here that explain why we're in very, very deep trouble around biotechnology. One is this very thin soup of an epistemology on which we're trying to construct our complicated society. The second is an absolutely astounding release of greed. When we have the coupling of a shaky social and values mechanism with a fierce engine of acquisition and possession, we get something very ugly. And that's what we're seeing in the biotech revolution. For example, between 1996 and 1998, we've seen the utter transformation of the basis of agriculture that has been around for thousands of years. And guess what? Nobody noticed!

I adore imagining conspiracies, and while I think there isn't actually much of a conspiracy out there in the biotech business, I also see that if you were to decide to design a conspiracy to dominate the world, the first thing to do would be to get control of the media, Well, that job has been done quite thoroughly. It is very, very difficult for heretical opinions to be expressed to the general and mainstream public. The next thing to do, if you were designing a worldwide conspiracy, would be to go ahead and take over agriculture, the means of feeding people. Then you would take over the pharmaceutical industry, change the way labor works on this planet, and start owning life forms. In fact, all of these changes are coming about quickly, conspiracy or not. And, since few people know about it, given the media monopoly, what will the public do about it?

Reading polls, even the polls the industry does, we see that when the right questions are put to people—such as "Do you want to know if there are genetically modified organisms in your food?"—an overwhelming, off-the-charts percentage of people say, "Yes." That encourages me. Ironically, it also encourages the biotech industry and the U.S. government, which supports the biotech industry, to do everything they can to maintain universal ignorance about what's going on.

Hiding the real issues

In one of the Council for Responsible Genetics' position papers, there is a critique of professional bioethicists whose job is to make new applications of genetic engineering desirable to the public. Will you describe this growing industry of bioethics and its ties to the media?

Yes. Bioethics is a profession in which people are paid money to render a defensible opinion about the ethics of new developments in biology. Well, he who pays the piper calls the tune. Truly, the question is, Under what auspices is the decision to be rendered? To whom are these people beholden? Who constructs the curricula? I'm not smearing all bioethicists. There are many people working in this area who are utterly sincere, uncorrupt, and independent. Yet one continually encounters people in this business who make pronouncements and turn out to be part of a system in which the subject of their judgment is constrained, a system in which their questions represent a particular point of view. There are some mechanisms, particularly around universities, that permit independent, ethical review of genetic engineering experimentation. I know some people who sit on these review committees for human experimentation and some are wonderful people, yet they have constraints in terms of what they can do. Obviously, it's not only appropriate but necessary for outside people to comment on the process and for independent media such as yours to make sure the public is able to enter into the conversation.

How do we turn attention to the real causes of systemic degradation?

The very ugly word here is commodification. Turning something into a commodity means transforming what we love and care about, and what we connect with in the world around us, into something that is an owned product, something that is fungible [interchangeable], something that is subject to an external control calling itself progress or science or whatever the slogan may be.

Biotechnology is presenting us with a wonderful opportunity right now to ask some deeply reflective questions. What is a human being? What is life? It may appear sophomoric, but these are not theoretical questions, these are real-life, on-the-lab-bench questions of science, and therefore actual questions of public policy, religion, morality, and ethics. We can ask how social agendas are built into biotechnology. We can ask, How can the public see that genetically engineered miracle crops can and are causing starvation? How can the public see and understand that the pursuit of biotech "miracle drugs" is also the pursuit of a particular kind of profit at the expense of some sick people?

We need to ask about the dangers. What will happen if even a few of our worst fears come true?

There are two approaches. One is that we have to have this kind of conversation loudly and publicly in schools and colleges and on street corners. People have to reclaim the connection to their own bodies, their own biology. Part of this conversation will also consist of reclaiming our language and images. So many of our daily metaphors are coming out of computers rather than out of living things. People are likely to find intimate humor in asides such as, "I woke up this morning with a crashed hard drive and booted up with an espresso." We should be using garden metaphors, not mechanistic language to describe our existence or the world.

The second approach, after deciding to talk with one another about these issues, is to be courageous. Years ago, I listened to a taped, public conversation between Daniel Ellsberg and Ram Dass on how to get rid of nuclear power and nuclear weapons. They speculated that the only way to get rid of them was a catastrophe. They imagined, well in advance, the significance of Three Mile Island and Chernobyl. Here are two extraordinarily decent and thoughtful people saying that maybe the only way humanity will learn is from a catastrophe! As people concerned about biogenetics, we need to have that same conversation. We need to ask about the dangers. What will happen if even a few of our worst fears come true? There are, after all, field trials going on right now that could let loose all kinds of nasty things. A fairly significant amount of work is going on in xenotransplantation, the crossing over of species lines between human beings and animals. These experiments run the risk of releasing pathogens into humanity that can't be stopped. I'm not saying this to be an alarmist—I don't think we serve any good by being alarmist—but how do we serve any good by dismissing dangers and refusing to face the realities?

What makes us human?

Biotech does offer us an opportunity to ask, What is a human being? What makes up what we cherish and love? It also poses the opportunity to see how the whole, living system works together.

You've said: "We should never let our rhetoric or our dreams cloud our assessment of the power and strength of our adversaries," and "Corporate accountability and citizen oversight are feasible." How do you see accountability and oversight coming about?

We always have a choice. We have a choice as activists to look at the power of a Monsanto, or a Time-Warner, and say, Here we are, scruffy and shrill, with no hope of obtaining resources that those corporate people command. Let's give it up. Or we can say, Let's be strategic. Let's level the playing field. Let's take these powers on. Our power is in the tremendous array of culture and history and human emotion that have not been commodified and cannot be commanded by our adversaries. The latter gives me immense hope for our ability to get a grip and turn things around. We have to be hard-nosed and practical, and not romanticized by our own rhetoric and siren song. A great model to follow is the Nestle boycott [of 1974–1984]. A group of people were extremely clearheaded and methodical in planning and executing that campaign with great precision and were hugely successful. They stayed clear and focused, and never abandoned their integrity.

Stealing genes

Will you speak to various projects, such as HUGO, that are now under way, and an emerging field of the medical industry often referred to as "biopiracy"?

Yes. There are a number of massive projects that deal with population genetics such as HUGO [Human Genome Organization, the organization of scientists working on the Human Genome Project], the Human Genome Diversity Project, and several derivative projects. All of these have certain characteristics. First, there are vast, rather extraordinary amounts of money involved in these projects, which is important to note because money gravitates to the greatest return on an investment. Second, all of these projects have commodification as their main agenda. There is a large amount of life patenting coming out of these projects. This means that while we are constantly told how scientists are doing innocent-sounding things like mapping our genes, they really are mapping in the sense that Columbus or Vasco da Gama mapped. They are methodically charting the territory that they will plant their flags on and make their own. In genetics, this bioinvasion means they are looking to own human genes so they can charge large numbers of us a lot of money for access to products that will make these bioimperialists very, very rich. Third, these projects represent the ultimate in cultural hegemony [dominance]—that is, a worldview from the rationalist, corporatized West that is being imposed on all of humanity at the genetic level. Finally, and particularly with the new environmental genome project, there is an agenda that appears to be eugenic in nature—that is, to wield ultimate power on the level of population genetics to redesign various physical traits and outcomes. In the real world this means gaining control of the human germline [genes that are passed on to offspring], the literal basis for who we are. Then these fellows, who evidently imagine they have the right to do this, will change humanity. They want to make changes that will be inherited, so that all succeeding generations of people fit not nature's design or God's design or what have you, but the design that emanates from the values of these almost unimaginably hubristic [prideful] scientists.

Much of this science makes judgments about individuals: who gets to be born and who doesn't and therefore what humanity looks like and consists of. Sometimes, when I'm speaking in public, scientists become irritated with me and say, You don't have the credentials to speak about science. You're not a scientist. And I say, Fine. If we're going to have the same ground rules, then you don't have the credentials to make judgments about moral, ethical, and spiritual matters. Show me how that was part of your training and background. Will you stay the heck out of those areas? Of course, if they did, they would have to close their labs. The very concept of genetic engineering science is totally infiltrated with a set of covert values and moral schema. These large-scale scientific/economic projects, carried out in public but in secret, imply some of the most extraordinary arrogance since Tamerlane or Genghis Khan.

Much of this science makes [moral] judgments about individuals: who gets to be born and who doesn't and therefore what humanity looks like and consists of.

The issue of biotech industry contracts with universities sets the deeper question we began with, which is, What kind of society are we creating? If it is common knowledge that today's educational institutions are deeply invested, literally and pedagogically, in the technical and commercial application of biological knowledge, where is public comment on this?

A respected professor is just now finishing research to document conflicts of interest between academia and industry. Even he, who designed this research, was stunned by the amount of conflict there is. Industry asked the same question you did, and they said, Let's get in there and get a piece of that action and make sure that we're in charge of what's happening.

My kids go to public schools in suburban Boston that are considered excellent, but I can say these schools are shockingly deficient. They are, basically, vocational schools. There's too little in them that I would call a decent liberal arts training. They're purely aimed at preparing children for the marketplace. The real liberal arts deficiency extends from questions of values, to questions of curriculum content, to homework assignments. The economic worldview permeates, saturates, everything that happens in these children's experience. We're turning out little worker bees, not engaged citizens, not thoughtful neighbors, and not loving human beings.

Invading the body

Will you speak to the controversies associated with DNA databanks?

Our government is very busily eroding our privacy on a genetic level with the proliferation of DNA databanks, some of which they mandate. The game is not only not over for those of us who want protection of our privacy, but it has gone far in the wrong direction, which is just now beginning to penetrate public consciousness. I'm receiving a lot of requests for information and interviews on DNA databanks. People ask, Isn't this a way to catch criminals? But this question is the criminal justice system's version of "we will feed the hungry" or "we will cure the sick"—myths sold by the biotech industry and their friends in government. They say, We will catch the bad people. How can you be against that? Phil Bereano, at the University of Washington and on the board of the ACLU, makes the point that we could also catch more bad people if we would say it's okay for the police to kick down our doors at will, or to stop us on the street and search us, or to open our mail. Are we willing to put up with absolutely anything to be more secure? Since the answer is no, we won't accept just any violation of our rights for the illusion or the actuality of greater security, then where do we draw the line? We have the Bill of Rights and the ACLU to help us figure out where to draw that line, and we ignore them at our peril.

As a society, we have fought very hard with very good reason to have certain safeguards for privacy and individual boundaries, and to constrain the criminal justice system. Now they're invading our bodies and our reproductive potential: our genes. The Fourth Amendment, which covers search and seizure, has been interpreted in many court cases as stopping at the skin. That's why fingerprints are permitted, even though they technically violate the Fourth Amendment. Specifically, fingerprints are allowed because they're an image of the outside of your body. The case law on this is amazingly explicit. But now there are DNA databanks. The last bastion of government resistance was the Massachusetts Supreme Court, and I happened to go and watch the court session on the case that now basically takes away the ability of certain citizens to keep the insides of their body private from their government. People argue with me, Well, we want to catch the bad guys. Okay! But we are also rapidly sliding down a very slippery slope.

They're invading our bodies and our reproductive potential: our genes.

Will you comment on the now famous 1990 case of John Moore's spleen, in which he lost rights to his spleen tissue because it had been removed from his body during surgery, and therefore lost any claim to its estimated one billion dollars' worth of derivative protein profit going to the University of California?

Yes, his doctor did real well. It's worth noting, though, that John Moore's claim was not privacy, it was theft. In other words, John Moore did not raise the issue that it's just plain wrong to do what was done to him. He wanted a piece of the action, saying his doctor had no right to alienate his body's tissues and not give him a share of the profits. I would raise different issues. John Moore is the person who was put through that horrible experience and I'm not making a judgment about him. But if they were, to use his phrase, "stealing" parts of my body, I'd want to talk about the right of another human being to do that. It's a very personal violation to take what is most essentially me and make it the property of another human being. In my theology, that's one definition of sin. I'd also want to talk about a supposed health care system that permits my doctor to take ownership of my body parts, or a government that allows and encourages companies to assert that they own life. Talk about sin.

People argue back and forth about organ transplants and different species' tissues being introduced to save or prolong life. Where do you make ethical decisions in this area?

I'm glad you asked that, because we're letting industry, with its particular agenda of profit, define the questions. They say, correctly, that 20 percent of people in the United States waiting for an organ transplant die before an organ becomes available. They follow that statement with, How can anyone be against xenotransplantation, or against other technologies that will save these lives? The answer is that there are more questions to be asked and possible answers to be found. Context matters, particularly the financial context—the profits at stake—for the person framing the ethical question about who gets organs and lives, and who doesn't get organs and dies.

Here are two examples of larger contexts. First, in Spain, virtually no one dies awaiting transplants because Spanish law maintains presumptive consent. You must affirmatively opt out of the transplant system if you don't want to have your organs donated after you die. In our country, you have to affirmatively opt in. Civil libertarians may take issue with presumptive consent, and surely it needs to be thought through, but organ availability was a policy decision, not a science decision, that solved transplant shortages in Spain. We have not had this conversation in our country—the issue hasn't been raised here. We haven't been given the opportunity to sit down with civil libertarians and say, What about presumptive consent? Is that an invasion? It's a solution that hasn't been put into the debate on xenotransplantation, though I assure you xenotransplantation experts know about it.

Second, there are people in the biotech industry talking about genetically engineering cows' milk so that it will resemble and replace human milk. They argue that women who are concerned about their breast milk being contaminated by PCBs [polychlorinated biphenyls] or PBBs [polybrominated biphenyls] or other environmental toxins out there can now feed their babies genetically engineered cows' milk that doesn't contain the nasty pollutants that could hurt their babies.

Over and over again, the wrong questions are asked and the wrong selection of solutions is presented to the public.

What about localized antibodies [defenses against disease provided by mothers' milk], and what about the bonding that occurs with breast feeding!?

Yes, there's a long list of "what abouts"! One of the "what abouts" is asking if any of the companies suggesting genetically engineered cows' milk are the same companies that have perpetrated the pollution that makes women's breast milk unsafe? Why not address the problem of polluted breast milk by dealing with the pollution? The reason is, of course, that businesses don't profit from reducing pollution. Over and over again, the wrong questions are asked and the wrong selection of solutions is presented to the public, to consumers. This is one of the primary problems activists have to address: reframing the questions so we are pursuing the right kinds of answers. Let's not buy into living in a world of narrow choices and debates that are framed by corporations and constrained by the images projected by well-paid public relations firms.

Will you describe the situation you've cited in Council for Responsible Genetics literature—that there have been two hundred documented cases of discrimination based on preexisting genetic conditions? Are we heading pell-mell into a society of "have and have-not genes"?

The figure of two hundred cases in our files refers only to our very tiny sample of reality. Society makes labels, and from those labels makes decisions. The real basis of discrimination is that certain characteristics are held to be a problem that should be tested for, and if it's a prenatal situation, then we are told to eliminate it; if it's a preemployment situation, we don't hire. One of the many problems with permitting genetic discrimination on the basis of labels is that we have no control over what will be the label du jour.

Right now we talk about people who have a certain kind of condition that we define as an "illness." People in the disability community often don't appreciate seeing their lives defined by what are seen by other people as limitations, much less hearing the medical establishment say, These are people who never should have been born, and we can help you to prevent more of these people from coming into being. Imagine the rich, full life of a person being reduced to one characteristic that is labeled, by powerful people external to them, as reason that they never should have been born! Furthermore, how well will society accept and support people whom they are told should never have been born in the first place?

The top of the slippery slope is preventing more cases of Tay-Sachs disease and the bottom of the slippery slope is "ethnic cleansing," or Kosovo. I've done a great deal of human rights work in my life, and a common denominator in many situations ranging from, say, South Africa to China is that they define the person they're about to oppress as differently human, and then subhuman. Human rights are those rights that accrue to anyone who is defined as human. Whether it's Kosovo or South African apartheid or a dictatorship in Chile, if you read the rhetoric of oppression, it's amazingly similar. The oppressors say those people are not quite human, not quite worthy in the same way as the ones generating the rhetoric.

Today we can see a situation of genetic apartheid, in which people are defined by some in the medical establishment who use unbelievably condescending rhetoric. "Genetic discrimination" is too gentle a term for the harm it does our sisters and brothers.

Worth, not usefulness

One of the values of the deep ecology movement is that it recognizes intrinsic rights and values across the board. In a world using deep ecology morality, we would no longer look at the value of a cow or a pig, or even an ear of corn, as merely valuable in terms of its usefulness.

Yes. I like to go past neutral terms, especially one like "rights"—which connects me with legal things and makes me shiver—to instead say "worth." It has to be okay for rational people in our society to talk in terms of value judgments, for that to be part of polite discourse instead of this pseudoscientific sham that we're all going to be legalistic and scientifically neutral—since we're not. It isn't just that another human being across the street or an ear of corn is okay, but that they have value, and that my connectedness to that other living thing is not neutral but an affiliation, an attraction to those things as other living beings in my world.

Beauty, too, is a much stronger force in our world than rights or even some kind of measurement of worth. Children all over are asking their parents, What about the shootings in these schools? What about Kosovo? It's important for adults to be able to give authentic responses to these kinds of questions. One of the things we can say is: When a mother who is wheeling her child in a carriage down the street stops and leans down and looks deeply into that child's face and touches its cheek, it doesn't make the six o'clock news. But those acts of deep love are continual among human beings and from human beings outward in the world—utterly continual and real and strong and present. They're not reported on "Dateline," or even in your fine publication. It's not how we experience the world and what we point at. But actually—and I don't think I'm a Pollyanna—we live in a world that is saturated in kindness and goodness that becomes invisible because we don't attend to it. We don't see it in the same way that we don't count the leaves on a tree. It's there and it's real. And by the way, it's something that can't be commodified, patented, or owned.

3

Genetically Modifying Food Crops Is Ethical

Ronald Bailey

Ronald Bailey is the science correspondent for Reason, *a magazine of politics, culture, and ideas. His books include* Ecoscam: The False Prophets of Ecological Apocalypse.

Genetically modifying food crops can increase their nutritional value and resistance to pests. Fears that genetically modified foods will harm human health or the environment are overblown and not supported by scientific evidence. Antibiotechnology activists' true goal is to have such foods not merely tested and labeled but banned, and their real target is not unsafe food but capitalism and globalization. By keeping genetically altered foods away from people who need them, these protesters may condemn millions to starvation or malnutrition-induced disease.

Ten thousand people were killed and 10 to 15 million left homeless when a cyclone slammed into India's eastern coastal state of Orissa in October 1999. In the aftermath, CARE and the Catholic Relief Society distributed a high-nutrition mixture of corn and soy meal provided by the U.S. Agency for International Development to thousands of hungry storm victims. Oddly, this humanitarian act elicited cries of outrage.

"We call on the government of India and the state government of Orissa to immediately withdraw the corn-soya blend from distribution," said Vandana Shiva, director of the New Delhi–based Research Foundation for Science, Technology, and Ecology. "The U.S. has been using the Orissa victims as guinea pigs for GM [genetically modified] products which have been rejected by consumers in the North, especially Europe." Shiva's organization had sent a sample of the food to a lab in the U.S. for testing to see if it contained any of the genetically improved corn and soy bean varieties grown by tens of thousands of farmers in the United States. Not surprisingly, it did.

"Vandana Shiva would rather have her people in India starve than eat bioengineered food," says C.S. Prakash, a professor of plant molecular genetics at Tuskegee University in Alabama. Per Pinstrup-Andersen, director general of the International Food Policy Research Institute, observes: "To accuse the U.S. of sending genetically modified food to Orissa in order to use the people there as guinea pigs is not only wrong; it is stupid. Worse than rhetoric, it's false. After all, the U.S. doesn't need to use Indians as guinea pigs, since millions of Americans have been eating genetically modified food for years now with no ill effects."

Shiva not only opposes the food aid but is also against "golden rice," a crop that could prevent blindness in half a million to 3 million poor children a year and alleviate vitamin A deficiency in some 250 million people in the developing world. By inserting three genes, two from daffodils and one from a bacterium, scientists at the Swiss Federal Institute of Technology created a variety of rice that produces the nutrient beta-carotene, the precursor to vitamin A. Agronomists [scientists who study crop production] at the International Rice Research Institute in the Philippines plan to crossbreed the variety, called "golden rice" because of the color produced by the beta-carotene, with well-adapted local varieties and distribute the resulting plants to farmers all over the developing world.

Can "green biotech" help the poor?

Last June, at a Capitol Hill seminar on biotechnology sponsored by the Congressional Hunger Center, Shiva airily dismissed golden rice by claiming that "just in the state of Bengal 150 greens which are rich in vitamin A are eaten and grown by the women." A visibly angry Martina Mc-Gloughlin, director of the biotechnology program at the University of California at Davis, said "Dr. Shiva's response reminds me of . . . Marie Antoinette, [who] suggested the peasants eat cake if they didn't have access to bread." Alexander Avery of the Hudson Institute's Center for Global Food Issues noted that nutritionists at UNICEF doubted it was physically possible to get enough vitamin A from the greens Shiva was recommending. Furthermore, it seems unlikely that poor women living in shanties in the heart of Calcutta could grow greens to feed their children.

The apparent willingness of biotechnology's opponents to sacrifice people for their cause disturbs scientists who are trying to help the world's poor. At the annual meeting of the American Association for the Advancement of Science last February, Ismail Serageldin, the director of the Consultative Group on International Agricultural Research, posed a challenge: "I ask opponents of biotechnology, do you want 2 to 3 million children a year to go blind and 1 million to die of vitamin A deficiency, just because you object to the way golden rice was created?"

Vandana Shiva is not alone in her disdain for biotechnology's potential to help the poor. Mae-Wan Ho, a reader in biology at London's Open University who advises another activist group, the Third World Network, also opposes golden rice. And according to a *New York Times* report on a biotechnology meeting held last March by the Organization for Economic Cooperation and Development, Benedikt Haerlin, head of Greenpeace's European anti-biotech campaign, "dismissed the importance of saving African and Asian lives at the risk of spreading a new science that he considered untested."

Shiva, Ho, and Haerlin are leaders in a growing global war against crop biotechnology, sometimes called "green biotech" (to distinguish it from medical biotechnology, known as "red biotech"). Gangs of anti-biotech vandals with cute monikers such as Cropatistas and Seeds of Resistance have ripped up scores of research plots in Europe and the U.S. The so-called Earth Liberation Front burned down a crop biotech lab at Michigan State University on New Year's Eve in 1999, destroying years of work and causing $400,000 in property damage. Anti-biotech lobbying groups have proliferated faster than bacteria in an agar-filled petri dish: In addition to Shiva's organization, the Third World Network, and Greenpeace, they include the Union of Concerned Scientists, the Institute for Agriculture and Trade Policy, the Institute of Science in Society, the Rural Advancement Foundation International, the Ralph Nader–founded Public Citizen, the Council for Responsible Genetics, the Institute for Food and Development Policy, and that venerable fount of biotech misinformation, Jeremy Rifkin's Foundation on Economic Trends. The left hasn't been this energized since the Vietnam War. But if the anti-biotech movement is successful, its victims will include the downtrodden people on whose behalf it claims to speak.

"We're in a war," said an activist at a protesters' gathering during the November 1999 World Trade Organization meeting in Seattle. "We're going to bury this first wave of biotech." He summed up the basic strategy pretty clearly: "The first battle is labeling. The second battle is banning it."

Later that week, during a standing-room-only "biosafety seminar" in the basement of a Seattle Methodist church, the ubiquitous Mae-Wan Ho declared, "This warfare against nature must end once and for all." Michael Fox, a vegetarian "bioethicist" from the Humane Society of the United States, sneered: "We are very clever little simians, aren't we? Manipulating the bases of life and thinking we're little gods." He added, "The only acceptable application of genetic engineering is to develop a genetically engineered form of birth control for our own species." This creepy declaration garnered rapturous applause from the assembled activists.

If the anti-biotech movement is successful, its victims will include the downtrodden people on whose behalf it claims to speak.

Despite its unattractive side, the global campaign against green biotech has had notable successes in recent years. Several leading food companies, including Gerber and Frito-Lay, have been cowed into declaring that they will not use genetically improved crops to make their products. Since 1997, the European Union has all but outlawed the growing and importing of biotech crops and food. In May 2000 some 60 countries signed the Biosafety Protocol, which mandates special labels for biotech foods and requires strict notification, documentation, and risk assessment procedures for biotech crops. Activists have launched a "Five-Year Freeze" campaign that calls for a worldwide moratorium on planting genetically enhanced crops.

For a while, it looked like the United States might resist the growing hysteria, but in December 1999 the Environmental Protection Agency announced that it was reviewing its approvals of biotech corn crops, imply-ing that it might ban the crops in the future. Last May the Food and Drug Administration, which until now has evaluated biotech foods solely on their objective characteristics, not on the basis of how they were pro-duced, said it would formulate special rules for reviewing and approving products with genetically modified ingredients. U.S. Rep. Dennis Kucinich (D-Ohio) has introduced a bill that would require warning labels on all biotech foods.

One scientific panel after another has concluded that biotech foods are safe to eat.

In October, news that a genetically modified corn variety called Star-Link that was approved only for animal feed had been inadvertently used in two brands of taco shells prompted recalls, front-page headlines, and anxious recriminations. Lost in the furor was the fact that there was little reason to believe the corn was unsafe for human consumption—only an implausible, unsubstantiated fear that it might cause allergic reactions. Even Aventis, the company which produced StarLink, agreed that it was a serious mistake to have accepted the EPA's approval for animal use only. Most proponents favor approving biotech crops only if they are deter-mined to be safe for human consumption.

To decide whether the uproar over green biotech is justified, you need to know a bit about how it works. Biologists and crop breeders can now select a specific useful gene from one species and splice it into an un-related species. Previously plant breeders were limited to introducing new genes through the time-consuming and inexact art of crossbreeding species that were fairly close relatives. For each cross, thousands of un-wanted genes would be introduced into a crop species. Years of "back-crossing"—breeding each new generation of hybrids with the original commercial variety over several generations—were needed to eliminate these unwanted genes so that only the useful genes and characteristics re-mained. The new methods are far more precise and efficient. The plants they produce are variously described as "transgenic," "genetically modi-fied," or "genetically engineered."

Plant breeders using biotechnology have accomplished a great deal in only a few years. For example, they have created a class of highly suc-cessful insect-resistant crops by incorporating toxin genes from the soil bacterium *Bacillus thuringiensis*. Farmers have sprayed *B.t.* spores on crops as an effective insecticide for decades. Now, thanks to some clever bio-technology, breeders have produced varieties of corn, cotton, and pota-toes that make their own insecticide. *B.t.* is toxic largely to destructive caterpillars such as the European corn borer and the cotton bollworm; it is not harmful to birds, fish, mammals, or people.

Another popular class of biotech crops incorporates an herbicide re-sistance gene, a technology that has been especially useful in soybeans. Farmers can spray herbicide on their fields to kill weeds without harming the crop plants. The most widely used herbicide is Monsanto's Roundup (glyphosate), which toxicologists regard as an environmentally benign chemical that degrades rapidly, days after being applied. Farmers who use "Roundup Ready" crops don't have to plow for weed control, which means there is far less soil erosion.

No dangers from GM foods

Biotech is the most rapidly adopted new farming technology in history. The first generation of biotech crops was approved by the EPA, the FDA, and the U.S. Department of Agriculture in 1995, and by 1999 transgenic varieties accounted for 33 percent of corn acreage, 50 percent of soybean acreage, and 55 percent of cotton acreage in the U.S. Worldwide, nearly 90 million acres of biotech crops were planted in 1999. With biotech corn, U.S. farmers have saved an estimated $200 million by avoiding extra cultivation and reducing insecticide spraying. U.S. cotton farmers have saved a similar amount and avoided spraying 2 million pounds of insecticides by switching to biotech varieties. Potato farmers, by one estimate, could avoid spraying nearly 3 million pounds of insecticides by adopting *B.t.* potatoes. Researchers estimate that *B.t.* corn has spared 33 million to 300 million bushels from voracious insects.

One scientific panel after another has concluded that biotech foods are safe to eat, and so has the FDA. Since 1995, tens of millions of Americans have been eating biotech crops. By 2000 it was estimated that 60 percent of the foods on U.S. grocery shelves are produced using ingredients from transgenic crops. In April 2000 a National Research Council panel issued a report that emphasized it could not find "any evidence suggesting that foods on the market today are unsafe to eat as a result of genetic modification." *Transgenic Plants and World Agriculture,* a report issued in July 2000 that was prepared under the auspices of seven scientific academies in the U.S. and other countries, strongly endorsed crop biotechnology, especially for poor farmers in the developing world. "To date," the report concluded, "over 30 million hectares of transgenic crops have been grown and no human health problems associated specifically with the ingestion of transgenic crops or their products have been identified." Both reports concurred that genetic engineering poses no more risks to human health or to the natural environment than does conventional plant breeding.

As U.C.-Davis biologist Martina McGloughlin remarked at the June 2000 Congressional Hunger Center seminar, the biotech foods "on our plates have been put through more thorough testing than conventional food ever has been subjected to." According to a report issued in April 2000 by the House Subcommittee on Basic Research, "No product of conventional plant breeding . . . could meet the data requirements imposed on biotechnology products by U.S. regulatory agencies. . . . Yet, these foods are widely and properly regarded as safe and beneficial by plant developers, regulators, and consumers." The report concluded that biotech crops are "at least as safe [as] and probably safer" than conventionally bred crops.

In opposition to these scientific conclusions, Mae-Wan Ho points to a study by Arpad Pusztai, a researcher at Scotland's Rowett Research Institute, that was published in the British medical journal *The Lancet* in October 1999. Pusztai found that rats fed one type of genetically modified potatoes (not a variety created for commercial use) developed immune system disorders and organ damage. *The Lancet's* editors, who published the study even though two of six reviewers rejected it, apparently were anxious to avoid the charge that they were muzzling a prominent biotech critic. But *The Lancet* also published a thorough critique, which concluded that Pusztai's experiments "were incomplete, included too few animals per diet group, and lacked controls such as a standard rodent diet. . . . Therefore the results are difficult to interpret and do not allow the conclusion that the genetic modification of potatoes accounts for adverse effects in animals." The Rowett Institute, which does mainly nutritional research, fired Pusztai on the grounds that he had publicized his results before they had been peer reviewed.

Activists are also fond of noting that the seed company Pioneer Hi-Bred produced a soybean variety that incorporated a gene—for a protein from Brazil nuts—that causes reactions in people who are allergic to nuts. The activists fail to mention that the soybean never got close to commercial release because Pioneer Hi-Bred checked it for allergenicity as part of its regular safety testing and immediately dropped the variety. The other side of the allergy coin is that biotech can remove allergens that naturally occur in foods such as nuts, potatoes, and tomatoes, making these foods safer.

Even if no hazards from genetically improved crops have been demonstrated, don't consumers have a right to know what they're eating? This seductive appeal to consumer rights has been a very effective public relations gambit for anti-biotech activists. If there's nothing wrong with biotech products, they ask, why don't seed companies, farmers, and food manufacturers agree to label them?

Under the "precautionary principle," regulators do not need to show scientifically that a biotech crop is unsafe before banning it.

The activists are being more than a bit disingenuous [insincere] here. Their scare tactics, including the use of ominous words such as *frankenfoods,* have created a climate in which many consumers would interpret labels on biotech products to mean that they were somehow more dangerous or less healthy than old-style foods. Biotech opponents hope labels would drive frightened consumers away from genetically modified foods and thus doom them. Then the activists could sit back and smugly declare that biotech products had failed the market test.

The biotech labeling campaign is a red herring anyway, because the U.S. Department of Agriculture planned to issue some 500 pages of regulations outlining what qualifies as "organic" foods by January, 2001. Among other things, the definition will require that organic foods not be produced using genetically modified crops. Thus consumers who want to avoid biotech products need only look for the "organic" label. Furthermore, there is no reason why conventional growers who believe they can sell more by avoiding genetically enhanced crops should not label their products accordingly, so long as they do not imply any health claims. The

FDA has begun to solicit public comments on ways to label foods that are not genetically enhanced without implying that they are superior to biotech foods.

It is interesting to note that several crop varieties popular with organic growers were created through mutations deliberately induced by breeders using radiation or chemicals. This method of modifying plant genomes is obviously a far cruder and more imprecise way of creating new varieties. Radiation and chemical mutagenesis is like using a sledgehammer instead of the scalpel of biotechnology. Incidentally, the FDA doesn't review these crop varieties produced by radiation or chemicals for safety, yet no one has dropped dead from eating them.

Labeling nonbiotech foods as such will not satisfy the activists whose goal is to force farmers, grain companies, and food manufacturers to segregate biotech crops from conventional crops. Such segregation would require a great deal of duplication in infrastructure, including separate grain silos, rail cars, ships, and production lines at factories and mills. The StarLink corn problem is just a small taste of how costly and troublesome segregating conventional from biotech crops would be. Some analysts estimate that segregation would add 10 percent to 30 percent to the prices of food without any increase in safety. Activists are fervently hoping that mandatory crop segregation will also lead to novel legal nightmares: If a soybean shipment is inadvertently "contaminated" with biotech soybeans, who is liable? If biotech corn pollen falls on an organic cornfield, can the organic farmer sue the biotech farmer? Trial lawyers must be salivating over the possibilities.

The activists' "pro-consumer" arguments can be turned back on them. Why should the majority of consumers pay for expensive crop segregation that they don't want? It seems reasonable that if some consumers want to avoid biotech crops, they should pay a premium, including the costs of segregation.

As the labeling fight continues in the United States, anti-biotech groups have achieved major successes elsewhere. The Biosafety Protocol negotiated in February 2000 in Montreal requires that all shipments of biotech crops, including grains and fresh foods, carry a label saying they "may contain living modified organisms." This international labeling requirement is clearly intended to force the segregation of conventional and biotech crops. The protocol was hailed by Greenpeace's Benedikt Haerlin as "a historic step towards protecting the environment and consumers from the dangers of genetic engineering."

Fears breed overreaction

Activists are demanding that the labeling provisions of the Biosafety Protocol be enforced immediately, even though the agreement says they don't apply until two years after the protocol takes effect. Vandana Shiva claims the food aid sent to Orissa after the October 1999 cyclone violated the Biosafety Protocol because it was unlabeled. Greenpeace cited the unratified Biosafety Protocol as a justification for stopping imports of American agricultural products into Brazil and Britain. "The recent agreement on the Biosafety Protocol in Montreal . . . means that governments can now refuse to accept imports of GM crops on the basis of the 'precautionary principle,'" said a February 2000 press release announcing that Greenpeace activists had boarded an American grain carrier delivering soybeans to Britain.

Under the "precautionary principle," regulators do not need to show scientifically that a biotech crop is unsafe before banning it; they need only assert that it has not been proved harmless. Enshrining the precautionary principle into international law is a major victory for biotech opponents. "They want to err on the side of caution not only when the evidence is not conclusive but when no evidence exists that would indicate harm is possible," observes Frances Smith, executive director of Consumer Alert.

The environmentalist case against biotech crops includes a lot of innuendo.

Model biosafety legislation proposed by the Third World Network goes even further than the Biosafety Protocol, covering all biotech organisms and requiring authorization "for all activities and for all GMOs [genetically modified organisms] and derived products." Under the model legislation, "the absence of scientific evidence or certainty does not preclude the decision makers from denying approval of the introduction of the GMO or derived products." Worse, under the model regulations "any adverse socio-economic effects must also be considered." If this provision is adopted, it would give traditional producers a veto over innovative competitors, the moral equivalent of letting candlemakers prevent the introduction of electric lighting.

Concerns about competition are one reason European governments have been so quick to oppose crop biotechnology. "EU [European Union] countries, with their heavily subsidized farming, view foreign agribusinesses as a competitive threat," Frances Smith writes. "With heavy subsidies and price supports, EU farmers see no need to improve productivity." In fact, biotech-boosted European agricultural productivity would be a fiscal disaster for the E.U., since it would increase already astronomical subsidy payments to European farmers.

The global campaign against green biotech received a public relations windfall on May 20, 1999, when *Nature* published a study by Cornell University researcher John Losey that found that Monarch butterfly caterpillars died when force-fed milkweed dusted with pollen from *B.t.* corn. Since then, at every anti-biotech demonstration, the public has been treated to flocks of activist women dressed fetchingly as Monarch butterflies. But when more-realistic field studies were conducted, researchers found that the alleged danger to Monarch caterpillars had been greatly exaggerated. Corn pollen is heavy and doesn't spread very far, and milkweed grows in many places aside from the margins of cornfields. In the wild, Monarch caterpillars apparently know better than to eat corn pollen on milkweed leaves.

Furthermore, *B.t.* crops mean that farmers don't have to indiscriminately spray their fields with insecticides, which kill beneficial as well as harmful insects. In fact, studies show that *B.t.* cornfields harbor higher numbers of beneficial insects such as lacewings and ladybugs than do conventional cornfields. James Cook, a biologist at Washington State University, points out that the population of Monarch butterflies has been increasing in recent years, precisely the time period in which *B.t.* corn has been widely planted. The fact is that pest-resistant crops are harmful mainly to target species—that is, exactly those insects that insist on eating them.

Never mind; we will see Monarchs on parade for a long time to come. Meanwhile, a spooked EPA has changed its rules governing the planting of *B.t.* corn, requiring farmers to plant non-*B.t.* corn near the borders of their fields so that *B.t.* pollen doesn't fall on any milkweed growing there. But even the EPA firmly rejects activist claims about the alleged harms caused by *B.t.* crops. "Prior to registration of the first *B.t.* plant pesticides in 1995," it said in response to a Greenpeace lawsuit, "EPA evaluated studies of potential effects on a wide variety of non-target organisms that might be exposed to the *B.t.* toxin, e.g., birds, fish, honeybees, ladybugs, lacewings, and earthworms. EPA concluded that these species were not harmed."

Another danger highlighted by anti-biotech activists is the possibility that transgenic crops will crossbreed with other plants. At the Congressional Hunger Center seminar, Mae-Wan Ho claimed that "GM-constructs are designed to invade genomes and to overcome natural species barriers." And that's not all. "Because of their highly mixed origins," she added, "GM-constructs tend to be unstable as well as invasive, and may be more likely to spread by horizontal gene transfer."

"Nonsense," says Tuskegee University biologist C.S. Prakash. "There is no scientific evidence at all for Ho's claims." Prakash points out that plant breeders specifically choose transgenic varieties that are highly stable since they want the genes that they've gone to the trouble and expense of introducing into a crop to stay there and do their work.

Ho also suggests that "GM genetic material" when eaten is far more likely to be taken up by human cells and bacteria than is "natural genetic material." Again, there is no scientific evidence for this claim. All genes from whatever source are made up of the same four DNA bases, and all undergo digestive degradation when eaten.

Will altered genes spread?

Biotech opponents also sketch scenarios in which transgenic crops foster superpests: weeds bolstered by transgenes for herbicide resistance or pesticide-proof bugs that proliferate in response to crops with enhanced chemical defenses. As McGloughlin notes, "The risk of gene flow is not specific to biotechnology. It applies equally well to herbicide resistant plants that have been developed through traditional breeding techniques." Even if an herbicide resistance gene did get into a weed species, most researchers agree that it would be unlikely to persist unless the weed were subjected to significant and continuing selection pressure—that is, sprayed regularly with a specific herbicide. And if a weed becomes resistant to one herbicide, it can be killed by another.

As for encouraging the evolution of pesticide-resistant insects, that already occurs with conventional spray pesticides. There is no scientific reason for singling out biotech plants. Cook, the Washington State University biologist, points out that crop scientists could handle growing pesticide resistance the same way they deal with resistance to infectious rusts in grains: Using conventional breeding techniques, they stack genes for resistance to a wide variety of evolving rusts. Similarly, he says, "it will be possible to deploy different *B.t.* genes or stack genes and thereby stay ahead of the ever-evolving pest populations."

The environmentalist case against biotech crops includes a lot of innuendo. "After GM sugar beet was harvested," Ho claimed at the Congressional Hunger Center seminar, "the GM genetic material persisted in the soil for at least two years and was taken up by soil bacteria." Recall that the *Bacillus thuringiensis* is a *soil bacterium*—its habitat is the soil. Organic farmers broadcast *B.t.* spores freely over their fields, hitting both target and nontarget species. If organic farms were tested, it's likely that *B.t.* residues would be found there as well; they apparently have not had any ill effects. Even the EPA has conceded, in its response to Greenpeace's lawsuit, that "there are no reports of any detrimental effects on the soil ecosystems from the use of *B.t.* crops."

As one tracks the war against green biotech, it becomes ever clearer that its leaders are not primarily concerned about safety. What they really hate is capitalism and globalization.

Given their concerns about the spread of transgenes, you might think biotech opponents would welcome innovations designed to keep them confined. Yet they became apoplectic when Delta Pine Land Co. and the U.S. Department of Agriculture announced the development of the Technology Protection System, a complex of three genes that makes seeds sterile by interfering with the development of plant embryos. TPS also gives biotech developers a way to protect their intellectual property: Since farmers couldn't save seeds for replanting, they would have to buy new seeds each year.

Because high-yielding hybrid seeds don't breed true, corn growers in the U.S. and Western Europe have been buying seed annually for decades. Thus TPS seeds wouldn't represent a big change in the way many American and European farmers do business. If farmers didn't want the advantages offered in the enhanced crops protected by TPS, they would be free to buy seeds without TPS. Similarly, seed companies could offer crops with transgenic traits that would be expressed only in the presence of chemical activators that farmers could choose to buy if they thought they were worth the extra money. Ultimately, the market would decide whether these innovations were valuable.

If anti-biotech activists really are concerned about gene flow, they should welcome such technologies. The pollen from crop plants incorporating TPS would create sterile seeds in any weed that it happened to crossbreed with, so that genes for traits such as herbicide resistance or drought tolerance couldn't be passed on.

This point escapes some biotech opponents. "The possibility that [TPS] may spread to surrounding food crops or to the natural environment is a serious one," writes Vandana Shiva in her recent book *Stolen Harvest.* "The gradual spread of sterility in seeding plants would result in a global catastrophe that could eventually wipe out higher life forms, including humans, from the planet." This dire scenario is not just implausible but biologically impossible: *TPS is a gene technology that causes sterility; that means, by definition, that it can't spread.*

Despite the clear advantages that TPS offers in preventing the gene flow that activists claim to be worried about, the Rural Advancement Foundation International quickly demonized TPS by dubbing it "Terminator Technology." RAFI warned that "if the Terminator Technology is widely utilized, it will give the multinational seed and agrochemical industry an unprecedented and extremely dangerous capacity to control the world's food supply." In 1998 farmers in the southern Indian state of Karnataka, urged on by Shiva and company, ripped up experimental plots of biotech crops owned by Monsanto in the mistaken belief that they were TPS plants. The protests prompted the Indian government to declare that it would not allow TPS crops to enter the country. That same year, 20 African countries declared their opposition to TPS at a U.N. Food and Agriculture Organization meeting. In the face of these protests, Monsanto, which had acquired the technology when it bought Delta Pine Land Co., declared that it would not develop TPS.

Even so, researchers have developed another clever technique to prevent transgenes from getting into weeds through crossbreeding. Chloroplasts (the little factories in plant cells that use sunlight to produce energy) have their own small sets of genes. Researchers can introduce the desired genes into chloroplasts instead of into cell nuclei where the majority of a plant's genes reside. The trick is that the pollen in most crop plants don't have chloroplasts, therefore it is impossible for a transgene confined to chloroplasts to be transferred through crossbreeding.

As one tracks the war against green biotech, it becomes ever clearer that its leaders are not primarily concerned about safety. What they really hate is capitalism and globalization. "It is not inevitable that corporations will control our lives and rule the world," writes Shiva in *Stolen Harvest.* In *Genetic Engineering: Dream or Nightmare?* (1999), Ho warns, "Genetic engineering biotechnology is an unprecedented intimate alliance between bad science and big business which will spell the end of humanity as we know it, and the world at large." The first nefarious step, according to Ho, will occur when the "food giants of the North" gain "control of the food supply of the South through exclusive rights to genetically engineered seeds."

Accordingly, anti-biotech activists oppose genetic patents. Greenpeace is running a "No Patents on Life" campaign that appeals to inchoate [vague] notions about the sacredness of life. Knowing that no patents means no investment, biotech opponents declare that corporations should not be able to "own" genes, since they are created by nature.

The exact rules for patenting biotechnology are still being worked out by international negotiators and the U.S. Patent and Trademark Office. But without getting into the arcane details, the fact is that discoverers and inventors don't "own" genes. A patent is a license granted for a limited time to encourage inventors and discoverers to disclose publicly their methods and findings. In exchange for disclosure, they get the right to exploit their discoveries for 20 years, after which anyone may use the knowledge and techniques they have produced. Patents aim to encourage an open system of technical knowledge.

"Biopiracy" is another charge that activists level at biotech seed companies. After prospecting for useful genes in indigenous crop varieties from developing countries, says Shiva, companies want to sell seeds incorporating those genes back to poor farmers. Never mind that the useful genes are stuck in inferior crop varieties, which means that poor farmers have no way of optimizing their benefits. Seed companies liberate the useful genes and put them into high-yielding varieties that can boost poor farmers' productivity.

Amusingly, the same woman who inveighs against "biopiracy" proudly claimed at the Congressional Hunger Center seminar that 160 varieties of kidney beans are grown in India. Shiva is obviously unaware that farmers in India are themselves "biopirates." Kidney beans were domesticated by the Aztecs and Incas in the Americas and brought to the Old World via the Spanish explorers. In response to Shiva, C.S. Prakash pointed out that very few of the crops grown in India today are indigenous. "Wheat, peanuts, and apples and everything else—the chiles that the Indians are so proud of," he noted, "came from outside. I say, thank God for the biopirates." Prakash condemned Shiva's efforts to create "a xenophobic type of mentality within our culture" based on the fear that "everybody is stealing all of our genetic material."

Offering more choices

If the activists are successful in their war against green biotech, it's the world's poor who will suffer most. The International Food Policy Research Institute estimates that global food production must increase by 40 percent in the next 20 years to meet the goal of a better and more varied diet for a world population of some 8 billion people. As biologist Richard Flavell concluded in a 1999 report to the IFPRI, "It would be unethical to condemn future generations to hunger by refusing to develop and apply a technology that can build on what our forefathers provided and can help produce adequate food for a world with almost 2 billion more people by 2020."

One way biotech crops can help poor farmers grow more food is by controlling parasitic weeds, an enormous problem in tropical countries. Cultivation cannot get rid of them, and farmers must abandon fields infested with them after a few growing seasons. Herbicide-resistant crops, which would make it possible to kill the weeds without damaging the cultivated plants, would be a great boon to such farmers.

By incorporating genes for proteins from viruses and bacteria, crops can be immunized against infectious diseases. The papaya mosaic virus had wiped out papaya farmers in Hawaii, but a new biotech variety of papaya incorporating a protein from the virus is immune to the disease. As a result, Hawaiian papaya orchards are producing again, and the virus-resistant variety is being made available to developing countries. Similarly, scientists at the Donald Danforth Plant Science Center in St. Louis are at work on a cassava variety that is immune to cassava mosaic virus, which killed half of Africa's cassava crop in 1998.

Another recent advance with enormous potential is the development of biotech crops that can thrive in acidic soils, a large proportion of which are located in the tropics. Aluminum toxicity in acidic soils reduces crop productivity by as much as 80 percent. Progress is even being made toward the Holy Grail of plant breeding, transferring the ability to fix nitrogen from legumes to grains. That achievement would greatly reduce the need for fertilizer. Biotech crops with genes for drought and salinity tolerance are also being developed. Further down the road, biologist Martina McGloughlin predicts, "we will be able to enhance other characteristics, such as growing seasons, stress tolerance, yields, geographic distribution, disease resistance, [and] shelf life."

Biotech crops can provide medicine as well as food.

Biotech crops can provide medicine as well as food. Biologists at the Boyce Thompson Institute for Plant Research at Cornell University recently reported success in preliminary tests with biotech potatoes that would immunize people against diseases. One protects against Norwalk virus, which causes diarrhea, and another might protect against the hepatitis B virus which afflicts 2 billion people. Plant-based vaccines would be especially useful for poor countries, which could manufacture and distribute medicines simply by having local farmers grow them.

Shiva and Ho rightly point to the inequities found in developing countries. They make the valid point that there is enough food today to provide an adequate diet for everyone if it were more equally distributed. They advocate land reform and microcredit to help poor farmers, improved infrastructure so farmers can get their crops to market, and an end to agricultural subsidies in rich countries that undercut the prices that poor farmers can demand.

Addressing these issues is important, but they are not arguments against green biotech. McGloughlin agrees that "the real issue is inequity in food distribution. Politics, culture, regional conflicts all contribute to the problem. Biotechnology isn't going to be a panacea for all the world's ills, but it can go a long way toward addressing the issues of inadequate nutrition and crop losses." Kenyan biologist Florence Wambugu argues that crop biotechnology has great potential to increase agricultural productivity in Africa without demanding big changes in local practices: A drought-tolerant seed will benefit farmers whether they live in Kansas or Kenya.

Yet opponents of crop biotechnology can't stand the fact that it will help developed countries first. New technologies, whether reaping machines in the 19th century or computers today, are always adopted by the rich before they become available to the poor. The fastest way to get a new technology to poor people is to speed up the product cycle so the technology can spread quickly. Slowing it down only means the poor will have to wait longer. If biotech crops catch on in the developed countries, the techniques to make them will become available throughout the world, and more researchers and companies will offer crops that appeal to farmers in developing countries.

Activists like Shiva subscribe to the candlemaker fallacy: If people begin to use electric lights, the candlemakers will go out of business, and they and their families will starve. This is a supremely condescending view of poor people. In order not to exacerbate inequality, Shiva and her allies want to stop technological progress. They romanticize the back-breaking lives that hundreds of millions of people are forced to live as they eke out a meager living off the land.

Per Pinstrup-Andersen of the International Food Policy Research Institute asked participants in the Congressional Hunger Center seminar to think about biotechnology from the perspective of people in developing countries: "We need to talk about the low-income farmer in West Africa who, on half an acre, maybe an acre of land, is trying to feed her five children in the face of recurrent droughts, recurrent insect attacks, recurrent plant diseases. For her, losing a crop may mean losing a child. Now, how can we sit here debating whether she should have access to a drought-tolerant crop variety? None of us at this table or in this room [has] the ethical right to force a particular technology upon anybody, but neither do we have the ethical right to block access to it. The poor farmer in West Africa doesn't have any time for philosophical arguments as to whether it should be organic farming or fertilizers or GM food. She is trying to feed her children. Let's help her by giving her access to all of the options. Let's make the choices available to the people who have to take the consequences."

4

Genetically Modifying Food Crops Is Not Ethical

Ralph Nader

Ralph Nader is an internationally known consumer advocate, lawyer, and author. He has founded many organizations, including the Public Interest Research Group (PIRG) and Public Citizen. His books include Taming the Giant Corporation *and* Who's Poisoning America. *He was a candidate for president of the United States in 2000.*

Spurred by corporate greed, the technology of genetic engineering is outpacing understanding in the sciences that underpin it. Selling genetically engineered foods is ethically questionable as long as they present threats of unknown magnitude to the environment and human health. Regulation of such foods by U.S. government agencies is weak, and most academics are too closely involved with industry to criticize it. Farmers and consumers, however, are becoming more wary of these products.

G enetic *engineering*—of food and other produces—has far outrun the *science* that must be its first governing discipline. Therein lies the peril, the risk, and the foolhardiness. Scientists who do not recognize this chasm may be practicing "corporate science" driven by sales, profits, proprietary secrets, and political influence-peddling.

Technology outpaces science

Good science is open, vigorously peer reviewed, and intolerant of commercial repression as it marches toward empirical truths. The rush of genetically engineered foods is leaving behind three areas of science: (1) ecology, often academically defined as the study of the distribution and abundance of organisms; (2) nutrition-disease dynamics; and (3) basic molecular genetics itself. The scientific understanding of the consequences of genetically altering organisms in ways not found in nature remains poor.

Without commensurate [matching] advances in these arenas, the wanton release of genetically engineered products is tantamount to flying

From the foreword, by Ralph Nader, to *Genetically Engineered Food: Changing the Nature of Nature,* edited by Martin Teitel and Kimberly A. Wilson. Copyright © 1999 by Council for Responsible Genetics. Reprinted by permission of Park Street Press.

blind. The infant science of ecology is underequipped to predict the complex interactions between engineered organisms and extant [existing] ones. As for any nutritional effects, our knowledge is also deeply inadequate.

Finally, our crude ability to alter the molecular genetics of organisms far outstrips our capacity to predict the consequences of these alterations, even at the molecular level. Foreign gene insertions may change the expression of other genes in ways that we cannot foresee. Moreover, . . . the very techniques used to effect the incorporation of foreign genetic material in traditional food plants may make those genes susceptible to further unwanted exchanges with other organisms. Still, the hubris [pride] of genetic engineers soars despite an enormously complex set of unknowns.

The wanton release of genetically engineered products is tantamount to flying blind.

Corporate promoters, such as the Monsanto corporation are racing to be first in their markets. Using crudely limited trial-and-error techniques, they are playing a guessing game with the environment of flora and fauna [plants and animals], with immensely intricate genetic organisms, and with, of course, their customers on farms and in grocery stores. This is why these marketeers cannot answer . . . many central questions. . . . They simply do not have the science yet with which to provide even preliminary answers.

Selective corporate engineering, unmindful of the need for a parallel development of our knowledge of consequences, can produce disasters. Costly errors involving past and current technologies—from motor vehicles to atomic power reactors and their waste products to antibiotic-resistant bacteria—should give us pause.

What are the proven benefits of genetically engineered foods that would offset these multifaceted risks? . . . Genetically modified foods "do not taste better, provide more nutrition, cost less, or look nicer." Why, then, would a person run the risk, however large or small it might be, of using them when safe alternatives are available?

Ineffective regulation

If the countercheck of science and scientists has been impeded for the time being by the biotechnology industry, what of other precautionary and oversight forces? On this score the record is also dismal. As the engine of massive research and development subsidies and technology transfers to this industry, the federal government has become the prime aider and abettor. In addition, the government has adopted an abdicating nonregulatory policy toward an industry most likely, as matters now stand, to modify the natural world in the twenty-first century. When it comes to biotechnology, the word in Washington is not regulation; rather it is "guidelines," and even then in the most dilatory [slow] and incomplete manner. On August 15, 1999, the *Washington Post* reported that the "Food and Drug Administration (FDA) is now five years behind in its promises to develop guidelines" for testing the allergy potential of genetically engi-

neered food. The Environmental Protection Agency (EPA) is similarly negligent. To quote the *Post* article again, "while the agency has promised to
spell out in detail what crop developers should do to ensure that their
gene-altered plants won't damage the environment it has failed to do so
for the past five years." *Post* reporter Rick Weiss then cited studies show-
ing adverse effects developing that the industry had not predicted.

The U.S. Department of Agriculture has been handing out tax dollars
to commercial corporations . . . in order to protect the intellectual property of biotechnology firms from some farmers. You can expect nothing
but continuing boosterism from that corner.

The creation of pervasive unknowns affecting billions of people and
the planet should invite, at least, a greater assumption of the burden of
proof by corporate instigators that their products are safe. Not for this industry. It even opposes disclosing its presence to consumers in the nation's food markets and restaurants. Against repeated opinion polls demanding the labeling of genetically engineered foods, these companies
have used their political power over the legislative and executive
branches of government to block the consumer's right to know and to
choose. This issue could soon become the industry's Achilles' heel.

---

*Selective corporate engineering, unmindful of the
need for a parallel development of our knowledge of
consequences, can produce disasters.*

What about universities and their molecular biologists? Can we expect
independent assessments from them? Unfortunately, with few exceptions,
they have been compromised by consulting complicities [involvements],
business partnerships, or fear. Although voices within the Academy are
beginning to be heard more often, both directly and through such organizations as the Council for Responsible Genetics, the din of the propa-
ganda, campaign money, media intimidation, and marketing machines is
still overwhelming. In 1990 Harvard Medical School graduate and author
Michael Crichton warned about the commercialization of molecular biology without federal regulation, without a coherent government policy,
and without watchdogs among scientists themselves. He said, "It is remarkable that nearly every scientist in genetics research is also engaged in
the commerce of biotechnology. There are no detached observers."

Consumers must be wary

There are more such observers now. The situation is changing. One sign
is how often Monsanto has to threaten product defamation lawsuits to si-
lence the media and critics, who, although being advised that such suits
would almost certainly fail in court, cannot easily absorb the expense to
get them dismissed. As bioengineered crops cover ever more millions of
acres from their start in 1996, the likelihood of side effects and unintended consequences looms larger. Farmers will realize they were not told
enough of the truth. And, as more foods containing genetic organisms
from other species enter the market, consumers will see there is no escape

other than to fight back and demand an open scientific process and response to persistent questions and miscues, with the burden of proof right on the companies. . . .

Consumers will see there is no escape other than to fight back.

For increasing numbers of people who want to eat, to learn, to think, and to act in concert as the sovereign people they aspire to be, the subject of an ever more wide-ranging bioengineered food supply must be subjected to a rigorous democratic process. As the ancient Roman adage put it: "Whatever touches all must be decided by all."

Food—its economic, cultural, environmental, and political contexts—is one of the ultimate commonwealths. The ownership and control of the seeds of life, through exclusive proprietary technology shielded by corporate privileges and immunities, cannot be permitted in any democracy. Commonwealths can neither be seized by dogmas of intellectual property nor can they abide the domination of narrow commercial imperatives driven by the lucre [monetary gain] and myopia [near sightedness] of wealthy short-term merchandisers in giant corporate garb.

5

Promoting Genetically Modified Crops in Developing Countries Is Ethical

Robert Paarlberg

Robert Paarlberg is an associate at the Weatherhead Center for International Affairs at Harvard University and a professor of political science at Wellesley College. He writes frequently on international agricultural and environmental policy. His special interests include food and population policy and environmental protection in Africa.

Questioning the safety of genetically modified food crops and the ethics of selling them is a luxury that only the developed world can afford. Developing countries have much to gain from adopting such crops, including increased farm productivity and reduced environmental pollution. They do face some risks, including limits imposed by seed companies' intellectual property rights, loss of biodiversity, and poor regulation due to weak governmental institutions. On balance, however, developing countries are likely to receive far more benefit than harm from the biotechnology revolution, and environmental activists are wrong to discourage these countries' acceptance of genetically engineered crops.

Today's agricultural revolution—especially the move toward transgenic or genetically modified (GM) crops—is being financed, commercialized, and (hotly) debated, mostly in Europe, the United States, and elsewhere within the rich industrial world. Yet it is in the developing world where the greatest human and environmental promise—or peril—of this new technology may lie. It is time to move the terms of the GM crop policy debate in the direction of developing countries' interests.

Farmers and consumers in the industrial world are already wealthy and well fed and can afford, if they wish, to take a highly skeptical, pre-

From "Promise of Peril?" by Robert Paarlberg, *Environment*, January 2000. Published by Heldref Publications, © 2000. Reprinted with permission from the Helen Dwight Reid Educational Foundation. 1319 Eighteenth St. NW, Washington, DC 20036-1802.

cautionary view toward this new technology. A majority of farmers and consumers in developing countries, on the other hand, are neither wealthy nor well fed, so for them precaution alone might not be appropriate. Governments and societies in the developing world also differ in their scientific and institutional capacity to manage these powerful new technologies safely. So even if developing countries have much more to gain from the GM revolution in farming, they may, at the same time, find it more challenging to pursue those gains safely and equitably.

Because of such fundamental differences, developing countries should not be asked or expected to "import" their agribiotechnology regulatory policies either from Europe or from the United States. The highly precautionary European approach might cost them too much in terms of lost farm productivity growth, while the industry-driven U.S. approach could put values such as equity or biosafety at risk. Rather than importing regulatory policies in this agribiotech area, what the developing countries need, most of all, is larger investment in their own indigenous scientific and institutional capacity, so they can shape this powerful new technology to suit their own distinctive local needs and circumstances.

The transgenic crop revolution: A rich-world phenomenon

GM crops have been grown commercially only since 1996, yet the area planted with GM crops has increased dramatically. In 1996, only 1.7 million hectares were planted with transgenic crops. By 1998, 27.8 million hectares were planted with transgenics (mostly herbicide tolerant soybeans and insect resistant maize and cotton). In 1999, 39.9 million hectares were planted with transgenics, a 44 percent increase in a single year.[1] By agricultural industry standards, this high rate of adoption is virtually unprecedented. Yet 99 percent of these commercial adoptions—by planted area—have so far taken place in just three countries: the United States (72 percent of the global area in 1999), Argentina (17 percent of the global area), and Canada (10 percent of the global area). Nine other countries were growing transgenic crops in 1999 (China, Australia, South Africa, Mexico, Spain, France, Portugal, Romania, and Ukraine), but with a combined acreage of just 1 percent of the global total.

The heated debate over how to regulate GM crops has also been, so far, mostly a rich country phenomenon.[2] The U.S. government has predictably sought to create a regulatory environment friendly to a further spread of the GM technologies and products being developed and grown so successfully by U.S.-based companies and U.S. farmers. Just as predictably, many European governments are taking a more skeptical view. For a number of vocal and visible activist groups in Europe (including environmental groups, food safety activists, protectionist farm interests, and critics of free trade and globalization), GM foods and crops are something to be resisted. A sharp policy conflict has thus emerged, mostly across the Atlantic, over what sorts of food safety, biosafety, or trade restrictions to place on GM crops or products; over what labeling standards to impose; and over what kinds of patent protection to permit. While the outcome of this policy conflict will doubtless be important to the fortunes of heavily invested agribiotech companies in the United States and Europe (such as Monsanto, Pioneer/Dupont, and Novartis), farmers and consumers in the rich industrial world may only be slightly affected in material terms, one way or another. Farmers in the United States and Europe will remain wealthy and prosperous and consumers will remain well fed—in many cases, overfed—with or without the further spread of transgenic crops.

Developing countries should not be asked or expected to "import" their agribiotechnology regulatory policies either from Europe or from the United States.

Farmers in the United States have developed a stake in GM technologies but not yet a vital stake. Most of the U.S. farmers currently planting transgenic seeds (including one-half of soybean farmers and one-third of corn growers) would remain commercially successful even if those seeds did not exist or if consumers stopped buying GM crops. U.S. farmers could stop planting GM seeds with little damage done. The highly competitive agribusiness sector in the United States could even adjust, in time, to a mandatory segregation and labeling of GM versus non-GM foods. Farmers and agribusiness firms in the United States may soon have to develop identity-preserved marketing channels in any case when a second generation of GM products—foods engineered to appeal to specialized consumer desires, such as those with higher vitamin or lower fat content—emerges.

For somewhat different reasons, the material stakes in the current GM food debate are also quite small in Europe.

There is no credible evidence of a food safety risk linked to any GM food currently on the market in Europe.[3] For many European opponents of GM foods, the issue is not basic health or wealth, or even environmental protection, but a post-traumatic stress syndrome regarding all food safety issues, following the recent bovine spongiform encephalitis [BSE or "mad cow disease"] crisis,[4] plus an effort to reassert "culinary sovereignty" in response to the hegemony of America's rootless—and tasteless—fast food culture. In France, a combination of farmers, labor unions, environmentalists, and communists have gone on the attack, not just against GM foods but also against McDonald's restaurants, imported beef grown with (non-GM) hormones, Coca-Cola, and various other perceived threats. In Britain, the Prince of Wales (a self-described organic farmer) has lent his prestige to the campaign, speaking out at the immorality of "playing God" by moving genes between species that could never breed naturally. All this is to be expected among consumers in wealthy, postmaterialist market economies. European consumers can afford to take a highly "precautionary" view toward the introduction of GM foods because they are more than adequately nourished without such foods. As for farmers in Europe, many can actually benefit slightly if GM crops grown in North America or Argentina are kept out of the European Union (EU) market or otherwise made unattractive to consumers with stigmatizing warning labels.

In the rich countries, then, the material stakes in the current agribiotech regulatory debate are no doubt high for the private companies developing the technology (and their shareholders) but surprisingly low for most farmers and consumers. The real stakeholders in the new GM crop revolution reside in today's poor countries. It is in the developing world that both farmers and consumers might realize sizable material gains, over their current circumstances, from the successful development of new applications from agribiotechnology. It is also in the developing world that some distinctive perils from this new agribiotechnology can be identified. These distinctive developing world circumstances—not the terms of the current trans-Atlantic debate—should be guiding the formation of agribiotechnology policy in most of Asia, Africa, and Latin America.

Distinctive gains from GM crops for developing countries

The Food and Agriculture Organization of the United Nations (FAO) has recently estimated that one in five citizens of the developing world—828 million people in all—still suffers from chronic undernourishment despite the dramatic gains in overall farm productivity in poor countries brought on by conventional (non-GM) plant breeding breakthroughs in the 1960s and 1970s, the so-called "Green Revolution."[5] The largest share of these still-malnourished citizens can be found in the remote and disadvantaged rural areas of Asia and sub-Saharan Africa that were bypassed by the Green Revolution. These areas were bypassed either because the soil, water, topography, and labor endowments were unsuited to the demanding set of farm management practices called for to make Green Revolution seed varieties perform (e.g., well-timed fertilization and irrigation and chemical pest control) or because the physical and institutional infrastructure to deliver fertilizers and chemicals—and low-interest credit—to poor farmers was missing.

Africa's disadvantaged farmers were those most obviously bypassed by the Green Revolution. Between 1970 and 1983, new, high-yielding rice varieties spread to about 50 percent of Asia's vast rice lands, but to only about 15 percent of rice lands in sub-Saharan Africa. Between 1970 and 1990, improved wheat varieties spread to more than 90 percent of planted acreage in Asia and Latin America but to only 59 percent of planted acreage in sub-Saharan Africa.[6] This goes a long way toward explaining why total agricultural production increased more than population growth in both East Asia and South Asia between 1970 and 1990 but fell behind population growth in sub-Saharan Africa, leaving an estimated 39 percent of all Africans undernourished by 1994–96, according to the FAO.

> *The real stakeholders in the new GM crop revolution reside in today's poor countries.*

The distinctive promise of the current GM revolution is that it depends less than the earlier Green Revolution on hard to get, hard to manage "packages" of purchased inputs. All the potential for enhanced productivity is contained in the seed of the new GM variety itself. Crop pests or diseases are managed not with purchased chemical inputs but through the genetically engineered traits of the plant itself, fully contained in the seed.

Tropical agriculture is technically more difficult than temperate zone agriculture because of poor soils, extremes of moisture, heat, and drought, and a plenitude of pests and parasites that attack animals and crops. Poor farmers in tropical Asia and Africa currently lose a large share of their crop (often more than 30 percent) to pathogens and pests. In some parts of Africa, draft animals cannot be used at all due to infectious or parasitic diseases. Here is where modern agribiotechnology carries special promise for the tropics: It makes possible the engineering of plants and animals (or the creation of animal vaccines) for very specific resistances to pathogens and pests. Poor (especially dryland) farmers in Asia and Africa also suffer low average crop yields in part due to nonbiotic stresses (such as salt or drought) on plants. Biotic and nonbiotic stresses are especially acute problems for farm animals in poor countries because feed quality and availability are low and veterinary services may be scarce or not affordable. The low productivity of animal agriculture in poor countries could be addressed by using both cellular and molecular agribiotech approaches to develop and propagate improved breeds, feeds, and vaccines. Farming is the most important source of income and sustenance for roughly three-quarters of all people in sub-Saharan Africa, so any farm productivity gains that come from a new GM revolution can produce welcome immediate gains for these poorest of the the world's poor.

Any farm productivity gains that come from a new GM revolution can produce welcome immediate gains for these poorest of the world's poor.

Consumers can benefit as well, not only from the development of micronutrient-rich GM crops (for example, rice engineered with enhanced vitamin A to counter eye damage among the poor) but also from GM varieties that could bring higher total yields.

If increased farm productivity from the use of transgenic varieties boosts food production and lowers the price of food staples in poor countries (especially in South Asia and Africa), the consumption of both food and nonfood goods among the poor would increase. This is because (unlike in rich countries) the price of basic food staples in Asia and Africa remains an important factor in total consumer welfare and overall economic growth. Only when gains in agricultural productivity in poor countries bring lower staple food prices can purchases of nonfood goods finally increase, and only then can the nonagricultural part of the economy finally start to grow.[7]

Two kinds of environmental gains might come from the development of GM crops in poor countries. First, pesticide use could be reduced (especially in Asia) through the spread of herbicide-resistant and pest-resistant GM varieties. In India today, excessive pesticide use on cotton has resulted in pest resistance to the chemicals and uncontrolled damage both to crops and the rural environment. Meanwhile, most U.S. farmers planting transgenic cotton with engineered pest resistance have been able to cut their sprayings from four to six per crop to zero.[8] Farmers in North America and Argentina today have enthusiastically adopted GM varieties, primarily because they help boost profits. Yet these new seeds also bring corollary environmental benefits in the form of less runoff of pesticides into surface and groundwater and reduced tillage. Second, natural rural ecosystems are under assault today in much of Asia and Africa due to a population-linked expansion of the land area devoted to low-productivity crop farming (especially shifting cultivation) and livestock grazing. If agribiotechnology could help farmers in these countries produce more food on land already in use, one result would be fewer additional trees cut, fewer watersheds damaged, less rangeland and hillside plowing, less soil lost, less habitat destroyed, and more biodiversity preserved.

Agribiotechnology research in rich countries might also provide valuable spillover benefit for conventional plant breeders in poor countries because transgenic crop improvements developed in labs in the industrial world can so easily be backcrossed into local crop varieties using ordinary, traditional breeding techniques. Indeed, it is the ease with which local breeders might take control of the valuable engineered traits that has inspired industry to search for various gene use restriction technologies, such as the so-called "terminator" technology.[9] In this respect, genetic engineering advances in rich countries can have positive rather than negative synergies with more traditional crop improvement efforts in poor countries.

Distinct risks for developing countries

It is in the nature of powerful technologies to carry significant potential costs as well as large potential benefits, and so it is for GM crops in the developing world. If transgenic seeds continue to be developed and commercialized exclusively by private firms, based on legal systems granting strict or exclusive intellectual property rights (IPRs), poor farmers may find these seeds too expensive to purchase. The seeds themselves may be "scale neutral" with regard to farm size. Yet if credit to purchase the seeds is available only to commercial farmers with significant holdings of high-potential land (or only to the politically connected) an initial result could be further marginalization of the poor.

GM seeds have the potential to offer much greater value to poor as well as rich farmers, but if seed company IPRs are defined and enforced in ways that prevent farmers from propagating the seeds for their own use on their own holdings (either through strict licensing or by the development of new restriction technologies), the result could be a significant increase in beginning-of-season fixed costs and cash restriction requirements. For poor farmers that have trouble getting credit, this burden may be enough to nullify the reduction in purchased input costs mentioned above. Some GM seed critics fear that poor farmers will be hurt by becoming dangerously "dependent" on the annual purchase of GM seeds. However, the greater danger is that they will never be in a position to purchase these seeds in the first place because they will be developed and commercialized by private companies that are mostly seeking to service the needs of successful commercial farmers on high-potential lands only.

In contrast to the earlier Green Revolution, which was developed by governments and philanthropic foundations and then delivered to farmers largely as a "public good," the current gene revolution is driven by profit-motivated private firms expecting to capture rents from their IPRs.[10]

This is not seen as a serious problem in the United States, where rules of patent protection that encourage private companies to invest in useful product innovations are accepted; where most of the companies in question are homegrown (such as Monsanto or Pioneer/Dupont); and where the full-time commercial farmers buying the GM seeds are generally wealthy, well educated, market-oriented, and politically well organized.

In developing countries, however, several distinct problems are associated with the private commercial nature of agribiotechnology. First, the private firms seeking to capture rents will naturally focus first on product innovations designed for use by wealthier farmers able to pay for the new seeds. This discourages needed investments in the "orphan crops" grown mostly by poor farmers, such as cassava, legumes, or sweet potatoes. This failing could be corrected through larger public investments by donor-funded national agricultural research systems in developing countries or through the Consultative Group on International Agricultural Research (CGIAR). Most governments in the developing world have long been stingy in making any agricultural research and development investments at all, however, and CGIAR is far behind the private sector in its basic capacity to develop transgenic varieties. CGIAR centers also know they would risk offending agribiotechnology critics in important donor countries in Europe if they were to attempt to promote research on GM crops.

Second, in developing countries private markets and companies (especially large multinational companies) and patent rights are often still a source of deep anxiety. Many developing countries party to the 1992 Convention on Biological Diversity have asserted that all indigenous germplasm should remain under "national sovereign control." Numerous developing countries have specifically excluded the practice of patenting plants and animals (as have most European countries under the European Patent Convention). Such nations are antagonized when private international companies employ U.S. patent law to gain property rights not just to plants but even to some of the smallest genomic components of those plants, such as expressed sequence tags. Further concerns are aroused by aggressive U.S. government efforts (through the Agreement on Trade-Related Aspects of Intellectual Property Rights in the World Trade Organization (WTO)) to link more general trade concessions to their recognition of plant patents, or at least link them to an alternative system of IPR such as the United Nations' convention called the Union for the Protection of New Varieties of Plants (UPOV).

In developing countries . . . several distinct problems are associated with the private commercial nature of agribiotechnology.

Many of the fears of these developing countries are overdrawn. Concentration within the global seed industry is still only moderate, with the 10 largest firms having 30 percent of global sales. The freedom of farmers to continue replicating their own traditional seed varieties on the farm would in no case be taken away. Still, the extension of U.S.-style patent law to plants and plant materials does threaten some of the free sharing of genetic information among researchers and breeders that was a hallmark of the earlier Green Revolution. U.S. patent law provides no "breeders' exemption" to permit further improvement of protected varieties (in contrast to the current UPOV) and offers no special "farmers' privilege" to resow seed harvested from protected varieties (as did the original UPOV, at least in practice). Particularly, when foreign-owned private companies seek exclusive patented ownership over processes to extract natural products long in use in the developing world (e.g., patents filed in the United States on processes to extract neem, a natural insecticide used in India for thousands of years), developing countries see reason to worry.

Tropical countries, aware of the importance and richness of their natural biological endowments, have also raised concerns about what GM seeds might do to increase the genetic uniformity of the crops grown within their borders. Genetic uniformity emerged as a concern in agriculture long before the GM crop era, when mechanization, commercialization, and plant breeders' rights all brought on a global narrowing of crops during the earlier Green Revolution. Transgenics are seen by some critics as pushing this decline in on-farm use of traditional varieties one step further. A much greater threat to biodiversity in poor countries comes, however, from a further loss of forest area to the continued spread of non-GM cropping, as is certain to accompany population growth if farming technologies are not upgraded.

While the new food safety risks possibly associated with GM foods have been a less prominent issue in developing countries . . . , biodiversity has been a more prominent issue.

While the new food safety risks possibly associated with GM foods have been a less prominent issue in developing countries than in Europe or Japan, biodiversity has been a more prominent issue. European-based environmental nongovernmental organizations (NGOs) have stressed the possibility of adverse impacts on rural ecosystems from transgenic varieties, including the potential for outcrossing to a wild relative species that might coexist with the GM crop. The hypothetical biohazards might include insect populations resistant to the toxins in Bt crops (that focus on a protein toxic to some insects) or the transfer of herbicide resistance traits from transgenic crops to sexually compatible wild relatives—resulting in herbicide-resistant "superweeds." In the United States, such hazards are contained well enough through safe and effectively terminated field testing under closely monitored conditions, using a mix of physical, biological, and temporal biosafety controls. In many developing countries, however, the capacity to undertake such testing may be absent.

This presents a difficult policy dilemma. The May 1999 report of the Nuffield Council on Bioethics resolves this dilemma as follows:

> The probable costs of the (mostly remote) environmental risks from GM crops to developing countries, even with no

controls, do not approach the probable gains of GM crops concentrated on the local and labor-intensive production of food staples. Are lower safety standards justified because, by producing more and better food and more jobs for the undernourished, or by reducing agrochemical use, GM crops save many more lives than they cost and improve lives than they worsen?[11]

Weak public institutions

In developed countries such as the United States, public institutions are generally well equipped to monitor and abate the social hazards that can accompany commercialization of a powerful new technology. In the United States, food crops with engineered genes are reviewed by the Food and Drug Administration for human food and animal feed safety and by the Animal and Plant Health Inspection Service within the U.S. Department of Agriculture for safety to agriculture and the farming environment. Crops with pest-resistance traits are also reviewed by the Environmental Protection Agency (EPA). The professional staff of these agencies carry out safety evaluations of industry-supplied data based upon regulatory policy and safety assessment approaches recommended by scientific expert panels. In developing countries, by contrast, public regulatory institutions generally lack a capacity to play this same testing and regulatory role. They are prone to oversights in monitoring and implementation and outright corruption by more powerful political or private sector (including corporate transnational) actors. Keenly aware of their own internal regulatory deficits, some governments in the developing world are opting to keep GM seeds out of their farming systems entirely. To avoid errors of underregulation, they may be making a mistake of overregulation.

As noted above, public institutions in the United States and elsewhere will soon face an additional challenge of developing identity-preserved marketing channels for agribiotechnology products to satisfy the strict labeling requirements that some affluent importing countries—including Japan and South Korea as well as the EU—are in the process of imposing. This step will be costly in the United States, but technically attainable and ultimately affordable. It is a step that will have to be taken anyway, given the anticipation of a second generation of even higher value GM food products targeted at distinct consumer preferences. For many poor developing countries, the creation and regulation of separate identity-preserved marketing channels, necessary for credible labeling, will not be technically possible or affordable. This implies that farmers in those countries could be excluded from the more lucrative international markets for GM products that might emerge in the years ahead.

Public institutions in many developing countries are also weak in their internal legal and political accountability. When public decisions are made regarding the regulation of agribiotechnology in the United States or Europe, a measure of accountability is ensured through institutions such as freedom of the press, democratic elections, institutionalized political access for stakeholders (including scientists as well as farmers, consumers, and industry), and the rule of law. In many developing countries, such institutions remain weak.

Policy choice in poor countries: An opportunity missed?

The distinctive mix of opportunities and risks has so far brought dramatically different policy reactions in different countries. In Latin America, while farmers from Argentina have been allowed to go full speed ahead with transgenic (herbicide-resistant) soybean production, in neighboring Brazil, NGO critics of GM crops have brought court cases that have, so far, blocked commercialization of transgenic varieties. In East Asia, while some countries, such as China, have sought to make full use of potential productivity gains from GM seeds, other countries, like Thailand, have recently succumbed to pressures from their customers in Europe and have announced that GM seeds will not be brought into their country until proven safe for human consumption.

One place where this haphazard process of country-by-country policy choice could go badly wrong is sub-Saharan Africa. In Africa, a free choice to participate in this new farm technology revolution is under threat of being denied. This denial of choice stems in roughly equal measure from the current actions of African governments, international donors, private industry, and environmental NGOs.

Many national governments in Africa are skeptical toward the GM revolution because it is coming to them through private firms that insist upon intellectual property rights. Yet these same governments continue to skimp on providing the public investments in agricultural research that are the obvious alternative to a market-led technology upgrade. African governments are also keeping out GM seeds because of a professed concern for the rural environment. Yet most have paid little attention to the rural devastation currently caused by expanding acreage under low-yielding, pest-vulnerable non-GM crops.

African voices are now being raised against the tendency of some GM seed critics from rich countries to keep the potential of the GM revolution out of Africa.

The cautious and stingy donor community (including bilateral assistance agencies in Europe, North America, and Japan and international financial institutions such as the World Bank) is also unwittingly reducing Africa's range of choice toward agribiotechnology. The donors have been eager to help Africans develop biosafety regulations on paper (modeled after the most expensive and demanding rich country practices), yet they have been slow to assist in building actual scientific and administrative capacity to implement such regulations. In many countries, the result has been regulation through a second-best strategy of import restraint.

Choices are also being denied when private industries (and the governments that defend them) insist upon IPR systems that deny on-farm seed multiplication options to poor farmers and restrict research options to Africa's conventional plant breeders. Extreme IPR demands such as these threaten to keep this new technology out of Africa entirely in the short run; in the longer run they could encourage a self-defeating (for the companies) piracy-based rather than legally contracted spread of GM seeds.

Environmental NGOs based in rich countries can also become a part of the choice-denial problem when they project onto Africa their own highly "precautionary" view toward this new technology. This is a view that farmers in Africa—who are not yet rich—can afford less well. While per capita food production and consumption have been growing recently in every other part of the developing world, they have recently been declining in Africa. The United Nations Food and Agriculture Organization forecasts that while the total number of chronically malnourished people will continue to fall in Asia and Latin America in the decades ahead, the total number of malnourished will increase sharply in Africa.[12] Since 1970, cereal yields (tons per hectare) in Africa have increased at one-half the rate seen in Asia, while population growth in Africa has remained much higher than in Asia. In some African countries, yields per hectare have actually fallen in recent years due to soil nutrient depletion (most African farmers use little or no fertilizer). Partly as a result, per capita consumption of basic foods (cereals, roots and tubers, and pulses) has tragically declined in East Africa by 9.3 percent.[13]

Africa needs an agricultural revolution, and African voices are now being raised against the tendency of some GM seed critics from rich countries to keep the potential of the GM revolution out of Africa. In Kenya, a new university based organization of biological scientists (calling themselves the "African Biotechnology Stakeholders Forum") recently wrote an open letter to policymakers in Kenya who have been holding back on allowing GM seeds into the country. This open letter presents the issue as one of scientific self-determination for Africa:

> In Africa, the realization that science and technology constitute the socio-economic and political power behind the industrial nations is still very much hidden. . . . Already industrial nations have perfected their biotechnology skills while Africa, on the other hand, has been made to be a mere observer and discussant of issues generated by nations in the North, some of whose agenda is to stifle the continent's acquisition and utilization of appropriate biotechnology, especially that which aims to produce food production. . . . Policy makers and those in a position to influence change and make a difference should understand and support policies that will best serve our national interest despite mounting attempts to curb the evolution and development of biotechnology in Africa. . . . There are signs that "global transfer" of crucial biotechnology skills and products to developing countries may soon slow down considerably if those in the industrialized countries continue to assume they know what is best for Kenya and the rest of Africa. This includes hindering rapid acquisition of various biotechnologies already possessed not only by developed nations, but also [some other developing nations], such as in Asia and Latin America.[14]

It would be unfortunate if the same environmental activists in rich countries, who previously waged an inspired and courageous battle to prevent the dumping of toxic wastes in developing countries, should now use their reputation to deny those same countries access to modern agribiotechnology. This is a powerful tool of science, not a toxic waste. It is the toxic quality of the current industrial world debate regarding GM seeds that the developing countries should perhaps choose not to import.

Notes

1. C. James, "Global Review of Commercialized Transgenic Crops: 1999," *ISAAA Report No. 12* (Ithaca, N.Y.: International Service for the Acquisition of Agri-Biotech Applications, 1999), vi.

2. L. Levidow, "Regulating Bt Maize in the United States and Europe: A Scientific-Cultural Comparison," *Environment*, December 1999, 10–22.

3. According to a May 1999 report from the U. K. Nuffield Council on Bioethics: "We have not been able to find any evidence of harm. We are satisfied that all products currently on the market have been rigorously screened by the regulatory authorities, that they continue to be monitored, and that no evidence of harm has been detected." See the Nuffield Council on Bioethics, *Genetically Modified Crops: The Ethical and Social Issues* (London, 1999), 126–27.

4. Over the course of this food safety scare, 40 people (all but one in Britain) eventually died from the fatal Creutzfeldt-Jakob disease, which has been linked to the consumption of meat tainted with BSE.

5. Food and Agricultural Organization of the United Nations, *The State of Food and Agriculture 1998* (Rome), 3.

6. J.R. Anderson, R.W. Herdt, and G.M. Scobie, *Science and Food: The CGIAR and Its Partners* (Washington, D.C.: World Bank, 1998); P. Pingali and P. Heisey, "Technological Opportunities for Sustaining Wheat Productivity Growth Toward 2020," *IFPRI 2020 Vision Brief 51* (Washington, D.C.: International Food Policy Research Institute, 1998).

7. K. Cleaver, *Rural Development Strategies for Poverty Reduction and Environmental Protection in Sub-Saharan Africa* (Washington D.C.: World Bank, 1997), 2.

8. C. James, "Global Status of Transgenic Crops in 1997," *International Service for the Acquisition of Agri-Biotech Applications (ISAAA) Brief No. 4* (Ithaca, N.Y.: ISAAA, 1997).

9. The "terminator" technology, originally patented by the Delta and Pine Land Company and the U.S. Department of Agriculture, ensured seeds from a harvested crop could not themselves be germinated. Monsanto, which subsequently gained ownership of this patent, never commercialized the terminator technology and made a promise in 1999, under heavy criticism, that it would never do so. See speech by Robert B. Shapiro, CEO, Monsanto Company, to Greenpeace Business Conference, London, 6 October 1999.

10. P. Pinstrup-Andersen and M.J. Cohen, "Modern Biotechnology for Food and Agriculture" (paper prepared for presentation at the international conference "Ensuring Food Security, Protecting the Environment, Reducing Poverty in Developing Countries," Washington, D.C.: World Bank, 21–22 October 1999).

11. Nuffield Council on Bioethics, note 3 above, 73.

12. Food and Agriculture Organization of the United Nations, *World Food Summit Technical Background Documents, Volume I* (Rome, 1996), 9.

13. J. Devries, "Rockefeller Foundation's Initiatives to Build Africa's Biotechnology" (background paper prepared for the "Regional Workshop on Biotechnology Assessment: Regimes and Experiences," organized by the African Centre for Technology Studies, Nairobi, Kenya, 27–29 September 1999).

14. "Re: Biotechnology and Kenya's Socio-Economic Survival," African Biotechnology Stakeholders Forum, Nairobi, Kenya, September 1999.

6

Promoting Genetically Modified Crops in Developing Countries Is Not Ethical

Miguel A. Altieri

Miguel A. Altieri is chair of the NGO Committee of the Washington, D.C. based Consultative Group of International Agricultural Research (CGIAR) and an associate professor of agroecology at the University of California, Berkeley. His books include Agroecology: The Science of Sustainable Agriculture.

Supporters of biotechnology say that genetically modified crops will help to feed the world and ease poverty, but this is not so. Even if such crops increase productivity, they will not cure hunger and poverty, which are caused by problems other than an insufficient world food supply. Furthermore, genetically modified crops threaten the environment, for example, by reducing biodiversity. Because there are better ways to improve agriculture in developing countries than to urge genetically modified crops on them, encouraging these countries to adopt such crops is unethical.

Most proponents of biotechnology portray genetically modified (GM) crops as hightech manna that will not only help feed the 840 million undernourished people in the world, but will also ease the poverty of the more than 1.3 billion who live on less than $1 per day. Biotech researchers promise new crop varieties that are drought tolerant, resistant to insects and weeds, and enhanced with vital nutrients such as vitamin A and iron. Increased agricultural productivity supposedly will reduce the costs of production and lead to lower food prices.

But before everyone rushes to embrace biotechnology as the solution to feeding the developing world, it is best to remember the maxim that if something seems too good to be true, it probably is. The putative benefits of GM crops may never become reality for the world's rural poor, especially since impoverished farmers will not be able to afford the seeds, which are patented by biotech corporations. Moreover, GM crops could devastate already fragile ecosystems by wiping out indigenous species of plants and insects that have thrived for centuries. This loss of biodiversity has serious implications for food security throughout the developing world: By planting fewer and fewer species of crops, farmers may increase the risk of famine since, in the future, those crops might prove vulnerable to changing climatic conditions or unforeseen diseases.

Although such scenarios have not yet come to pass, GM crops are already eroding food security in the developing world. The seduction of biotechnology has begun to divert public attention and precious resources from more reliable methods of increasing agricultural productivity—proven agroecological techniques that will not only enhance the livelihood of the rural poor, but that will preserve the environment.

Reality check

Biotech advocates who argue that GM crops are the solution to world hunger tend to overlook the real problem. We are constantly bombarded with statistics implying that food production is failing to keep pace with a global population that is growing by an estimated 77 million people each year. This statistical bombardment persists despite the absence of a proven relationship between the prevalence of hunger in a given country and the density of its population. For every densely populated and hungry nation such as Bangladesh or Haiti, there is a sparsely populated and hungry nation such as Brazil or Indonesia. Indeed, between the late 1960s and the early 1990s, the number of undernourished people fell by only 80 million, even as the amount of food available per capita increased and global food prices declined.

Poverty is the key reason why 840 million people (most of whom live in the developing world) do not have enough to eat. At present, hunger is not a matter of agricultural limits but a problem of masses of people not having sufficient access to food or the means to produce it. At most, biotechnology has the yet-unrealized potential to improve the quality of and increase the quantity of food—but there is no guarantee that this food will be made available to those who need it most.

Before everyone rushes to embrace biotechnology as the solution to feeding the developing world, it is best to remember the maxim that if something seems too good to be true, it probably is.

In the last 25 years, enough food was produced to feed everyone in the world, had that food been more evenly shared. But the truth is that there is no global mechanism in place to undertake such a massive redistribution. Instead, food is rushing to countries that already have more than enough to eat. Developing nations with swelling populations need to become truly self-sufficient. In order to achieve this goal, they must increase food production by improving their domestic agricultural systems. However, this task is constrained by considerable environmental obstacles. An estimated 850 million people live on land threatened by desertification. Another 500 million reside on terrain that is too steep to cultivate. Most of the rural poor live in the latitudinal band between the Tropic of Cancer and the Tropic of Capricorn, the region that will be most vulnerable to the effects of global warming.

Biotech researchers pledge to counter problems associated with food production and distribution by developing GM crops with traits considered desirable by small farmers, such as enhanced competitiveness against weeds and drought tolerance. These new attributes, however, would not necessarily be a panacea. Traits such as drought tolerance are polygenic, which means they are determined by the interaction of multiple genes. Consequently, the development of crops with such traits is a complex process that could take at least 10 years. And under these circumstances, genetic engineering does not give you something for nothing. When you tinker with multiple genes to create a desired trait, you inevitably end up sacrificing other traits, such as productivity. As a result, use of a drought-tolerant plant would boost crop yields by only 30 to 40 percent. Any additional yield increases would have to come from improved environmental practices (such as enhancing soil cover for improved water retention) rather than from the genetic manipulation of specific characteristics.

Even if biotechnology contributes to increased crop harvests, poverty will not necessarily decline.

Even if biotechnology contributes to increased crop harvests, poverty will not necessarily decline. Many poor farmers in developing countries do not have access to cash, credit, technical assistance, or markets. The so-called Green Revolution of the 1950s and 1960s bypassed such farmers because planting the new high-yield crops and maintaining them through the use of pesticides and fertilizers was too costly for impoverished landowners. Data show that, in both Asia and Latin America, wealthy farmers with larger and better-endowed lands gained the most from the Green Revolution, whereas farmers with fewer resources often gained little. The "Gene Revolution" might only end up repeating the mistakes of its predecessor. Genetically modified seeds are under corporate control and patent protection; consequently, they are very expensive. Since many developing countries still lack the institutional infrastructure and low-interest credit necessary to deliver these new seeds to poor farmers, biotechnology will only exacerbate marginalization.

Moreover, poor farmers do not fit into the marketing niche of private corporations, which focus on biotechnological innovations for the commercial-agricultural sectors of industrial and developing nations, where these corporations expect a huge return on their research investment. The private sector often ignores important crops such as cassava, which is a staple for 500 million people worldwide. The few impoverished landowners who will have access to biotechnology will become dangerously dependent on the annual purchase of genetically modified seeds.

These farmers will have to abide by onerous intellectual property agreements not to plant seeds yielded from a harvest of bioengineered plants. Such stipulations are an affront to traditional farmers, who for centuries have saved and shared seeds as part of their cultural legacy. Some scientists and policy makers suggest that large investments through public-private partnerships can help developing countries acquire the indigenous scientific and institutional capacity to shape biotechnology to suit the needs and circumstances of small farmers. But once again, corporate intellectual property rights to genes and gene-cloning technology might play spoiler. For instance, Brazil must negotiate license agreements with nine different companies before a virus-resistant papaya developed with researchers at Cornell University can be released to poor farmers.

An environmental time bomb

Biotechnology threatens to exacerbate environmental problems in the developing world. The marketing strategy of biotech corporations is to create broad international seed markets for a single commodity—a practice that tends to foster genetic homogeneity. Although some degree of crop uniformity may have certain economic advantages, it has serious ecological drawbacks. History has shown that a huge area planted with a single crop species is highly vulnerable to changing climatic conditions or the emergence of a new, matching strain of a pathogen or pest. For instance, all of the potatoes planted in 19th-century Ireland were descendants of just two genetic varieties, both of which lacked resistance to the blight that plunged the country into famine. Similarly, in the 1970s, Soviet farmers planted 40 million hectares with a new variety of a so-called miracle grain that, despite careful testing, proved unable to survive Russia's harsh winters. In the developing world, many native crop species are resistant to pests, adapt well to marginal environments, and allow farmers to cope with varying climates. The widespread planting of a single crop species leads to a loss of genetic diversity that reduces the options for farmers in the future.

Today's miracle crops may be the progenitors of tomorrow's invasive species.

Biotech crops pose a threat to biodiversity not only by crowding out indigenous species, but by breeding with them. The transfer of genetic traits from crops to other related species through the spread of pollen and seeds is always a concern. But in the developing world, where many countries constitute centers of genetic diversity (tropical forests alone host as much as 90 percent of the world's species), crossbreeding is likely to occur more frequently and with more serious consequences. An environmental group in Chile warns that genetically modified potatoes could contaminate 165 indigenous potato crops grown on Chiloe Island by Huilliche Indians. Especially worrisome is the possibility that GM crops—endowed with traits such as resistance to viruses, insects, and herbicides—might pass those characteristics along to wild relatives, thereby creating "superweeds" that will proliferate in farmers' fields. Today's miracle crops may be the progenitors of tomorrow's invasive species.

Another example of how the development of "beneficial" traits can backfire is the case of Bt corn—which uses a gene derived from the *Bacillus thuringiensis* bacterium to produce a substance specifically toxic to corn borers. But such a substance might be lethal to other insects. A recent European laboratory study demonstrated that the mortality rate of the green lacewing (an insect that preys on crop pests such as aphids) increased by two thirds after it ingested insects that had fed on Bt corn. Ecologists have also discovered that the Bt toxin remains active in the soil for at least 234 days after the crop is plowed under. The Bt toxin can kill important soil organisms, affecting processes such as the breakdown of organic matter, which is essential to soil fertility. This discovery is of serious concern to most poor farmers who cannot purchase expensive chemical fertilizers but who must rely instead on local organic inputs for crop nutrition.

A better solution

Alternatives to reinventing agriculture through biotechnology already exist in the developing world. A perfect example is the problem of vitamin A deficiency, which threatens the health of as many as 250 million children worldwide. Genetically modified rice capable of producing vitamin A is being heralded by the biotech community as the best hope for these children. But food preferences in rural areas of the developing world are culturally determined, and it is unlikely that Asians will consume this "orange rice" while traditional white rice is plentiful. Providing a rich alternative source of vitamin A, both wild and cultivated leafy greens grow in abundance in and around paddy rice fields. Although these greens are peripheral to the diet of the peasant household, many peasant communities gather them to supplement family nutrition and income. Lack of awareness is often the key reason why these vitamin-rich vegetables do not play more of a role in the family diet throughout the developing world. Ironically, biotechnology threatens the viability of these leafy green plants. Because some GM crops are resistant to weed-killing herbicides, farmers are inclined to spray large amounts of chemicals, such as glyphosate, that kill all plants except the genetically modified ones.

Much of the food needed in the developing world can be produced by small farmers using "agroecological" technologies, which foster self-reliance and protect the environment. Agroecology emphasizes the conservation of vital resources (soil, water, and financial capital), the use of natural inputs (such as organic fertilizers) instead of synthetic toxic products, the diversification of crops, and social processes that emphasize community participation and empowerment. For example, in Central America, thousands of hillside farmers are using the bean *Mucuna deeringiana* ("velvet bean") as "green manure"—a term to describe a crop that is plowed under to act as fertilizer. Green manure crops provide large quantities of nitrogen for soil, protect the land from wind and water erosion, and even provide a potential source of fodder to be sold or fed to animals. But unlike chemical fertilizers, they are nontoxic, inexpensive, and self-sustaining. Central American farmers who have integrated green manure into their soil have more than doubled corn production while conserving topsoil—even amid the destruction wrought by Hurricane Mitch in 1998.

Such approaches, now being spearheaded by farmers' groups and nongovernmental organizations throughout the developing world, are already making a significant contribution to food security at household, national, and regional levels in Africa, Asia, and Latin America. Increasing the agricultural productivity of small landowners not only expands food supplies, but reduces poverty among the people who are perpetually denied the benefits of the "new-and-improved" agricultural technologies periodically introduced to the developing world. A failure to promote such people-centered agricultural research and development by diverting funds and expertise to biotechnology will foreclose on a historic opportunity to increase agricultural productivity in environmentally benign and socially uplifting ways.

7

Altering Human Genes Is Ethical

Gregory Stock and John Campbell
(panel discussion)

Gregory Stock and John Campbell, both professors at the School of Medicine of the University of California, Los Angeles, were organizers of a March 1998 symposium on human germline genetic engineering at which the panel discussion excerpted here took place. James D. Watson is codiscoverer of the structure of DNA, a winner of the 1962 Nobel Prize in Medicine, president of Cold Spring Harbor Laboratory, and was from 1988 to 1992 the head of the United States part of the Human Genome Project. John Fletcher is Kornfeld Professor of Biomedical Ethics at the University of Virginia. Andrea Bonnicksen is a professor in the Political Science Department at Northern Illinois University. Leroy Hood is the inventor of the gene sequencing machine that has helped to make possible the deciphering of the human and other genomes and is the founding chair of the Department of Molecular Biotechnology at the University of Washington. Lee M. Silver, a professor specializing in mammalian genetics at Princeton University, is the author of Remaking Eden, *a book that presents a positive view of genetic engineering of humans. Michael R. Rose is a professor at the University of California, Irvine, and a specialist in human aging. Daniel Koshland Jr., is a professor at the University of California, Berkeley, and was editor of* Science *magazine from 1985 to 1995.*

Modifying germline genes—those that can be passed on to offspring—will allow the genes that cause inherited diseases to be removed from a family's collection of genes. Far from being unethical, germline genetic engineering will enable science to improve the poor genetic allotment that evolution gives to some individuals. This technology should be developed carefully, beginning with animal experiments, but it should not be excessively regulated. There is no reason not to change the human genome, and indeed, the possibility of humans being able to direct the evolution of their own species is exciting.

James D. Watson: . . . This is the first gathering where people have talked openly about germline [genetic] engineering [of humans]. Partly, it was in order to get somatic [gene] therapy going that it was said, "Well, we're not doing germline. That is bad. But somatic is not bad morally." It virtually implied there was a moral decision to make about germline, as if it was some great Rubicon [turning point or dividing line] and involved going against natural law. I've indicated, I think, that there is no basis for this view.

So, we are fighting the statement that somatic is safe, therefore, germline is unsafe; whereas, in fact, if anything is going to save us, if we need to be saved someday, it's going to be germline engineering.

Future experiments

Gregory Stock: Dr. Watson, you had a large part in creating or making successful the Human Genome Project. . . .

James D. Watson: No. No. Lee Hood. He got the [gene sequencing] machine. Without him the sequence of the human genome would be just hot air.

Gregory Stock: Well, Lee Hood may have made it work, . . . but you were certainly involved in some *small* way. What I wanted to ask is this: If there is no Rubicon to cross with germline engineering, and some approaches have a greater possibility of success than others, is human germline work something we then need to be thinking about trying—at least at a research level—to see whether there are possibilities worth realizing? Should there be some sort of a project toward this goal?

James D. Watson: Well, I wouldn't make it difficult to do the experiments, which is what the proposed laws against human cloning would have done. [Those laws] could make it very difficult to do . . . experiments . . . on homologous recombination, which is simply "correcting" a gene. We've got to be very careful not to admit at the outset that we're three-quarters evil and a quarter good. I just don't see the evil nature of what we're trying to do.

If anything is going to save us, if we need to be saved someday, it's going to be germline engineering.

Genetics, in many people's eyes, has a bad connotation of the State or others determining people's lives. Which is why, again, the State should stay out of it. My feeling is, the State shouldn't tell a person either to have it or not to have it. If the procedures work people will use them, and if they don't work or if it's dangerous, it will stop.

The real enemy is a preexisting genetic inequality which makes some people unable to function well in the world. Terrible diseases—that's the enemy. Whereas some people are convinced the enemy is the people who study the genes, that we are evil people. I don't think we're any more evil than the people who run this Music Department. You know? I don't know if we're better or worse. And I suspect we're deep down trying to respond to a long-term need, and the music people are making us happy by singing hymns, which cheers us up. We should be proud of what we're doing and not worry about whether we're destroying the genetic patri-mony of the world, which is awfully cruel to too many people. And I think that that's what we're all trying to fight. . . . I'm sure I will be mis-quoted by someone who says I'm gung ho to go ahead and do it [human germline engineering]. I would do it if it made someone's life better. We get a lot of pleasure from helping other people. That's what we're trying to do.

Gregory Stock: Thank you.

John Fletcher: Since we are talking about regulation, I'd like briefly to review what university-based or industry-based scientists need to know.

Somatic-cell [gene] transfer research in humans is now regulated, in all of its phases, by the Food and Drug Administration [FDA]. What about crossing the line to human germline gene transfer experiments? The Na-tional Institutes of Health (NIH)'s Recombinant Advisory Committee's [NIH-RAC] policy on intentional germline transfer is that it "will not now entertain" protocols [experiment plans] with this aim. Obviously, much more research in animals must occur, as well as public discussion, to cross this line. Since germline gene transfer experiments will occur in gametes or embryos, the one area to watch carefully is research with embryoni-cally derived stem cells. In 1994 Congress prohibited federal funding of any research that would harm human embryos. But this ban does not ap-ply to privately funded research.

We face not a slope but a course of action with stopping points and places to draw lines.

If your research is privately funded, there are no federal legal barriers to deriving stem cells from embryos. One needs to know if state law per-mits this research, before submitting a protocol for the research to the In-stitutional Review Board [IRB]. If your institution has signed a Multiple Project Assurance with the Office of Protection from Research Risks at the NIH, you promise to abide by the regulations to protect human subjects, no matter the source of funding. The "protection of human subjects" is-sues do not apply to embryos, but to the persons who are sources of em-bryos to be used experimentally. The privacy of couples in infertility treatment or donors of gametes [egg or sperm cells] needs to be protected. A process of informed consent for donating embryos or gametes for re-search needs review and approval. Finally, there are some ethical consid-erations about the outer limits (14 days) of permissible embryo research and prohibiting any future uses of research embryos for implantation. The report of the NIH Human Embryo Research Panel and the British guidelines for embryo research provide guidance on these points. The im-portant message for local IRBs is that it is not illegal to do privately funded embryo research, as long as the personnel, facilities, and equip-ment to be involved in this research are not substantially subsidized by federal funding. Research that involves putting genes into human cells or embryos requires the approval of the NIH-RAC and would also be regu-lated by the FDA.

John Campbell: Most of the research I envisage being done in the next five or ten years would be animal work. So, even if there was a prohibition on actually putting genes in human cells, it would not be decisive in inhibiting the research that needs to be done.

How dangerous are gene changes?

Gregory Stock: Dr. Watson dismissed the slippery-slope argument, the argument some people make that, if we once start to do these things [alter human genes], then gradually we will go down to who knows where. It has always seemed to me that either we're already on that slippery slope, and so might as well forget about it, or that it doesn't exist. Does anybody have any thoughts about the nature of the sort of reinforcement and self-reinforcement that occurs with these kinds of developments?

Andrea Bonnicksen: I would like to suggest a couple of other metaphors for the slippery slope that I've seen in the literature. One is to talk about us rapelling down the slope—that is, rather than just slipping on down without any stopping point, we can rapel from the building back and forth with stopping points. Another metaphor is that of the ramshackle staircase: instead of sliding down the slope, we instead are going down a rickety kind of staircase, and at points we stop and look back and fix it, and then we keep going. These metaphors suggest that—with these new techniques—we face not a slope but a course of action with stopping points and places to draw lines.

Gregory Stock: Lee, did you have a comment to make?

Leroy Hood: I related to this idea of the sanctity of the human germline. Remember, each of our chromosomes differs by 1 letter of the DNA language in every 500. And each of our chromosomes, when it goes through the necessary manipulations to make sperm, actually undergoes recombinational events where the information is scrambled. Indeed, there are an enormous number of other events where information is altered, is rearranged, and is changed.

I would reject, utterly, the idea of a slippery slope, because it seems to be arguing that we're doing something unnatural. In fact, it is quite the contrary. We're using exactly the same kinds of techniques used by evolution, but what we're attempting to do, in a thoughtful and rational way, is to facilitate evolution, so it doesn't operate in a blind fashion—most of the changes being neutral or deleterious—but in an optimizing fashion. It's exactly the same as the analogy for antibiotics. You could argue that maybe some human would someday run into the fungus that made penicillin, but on the other hand is it unnatural? Is it a slippery slope to manipulate molecules that could kill bacteria?

The other point I would make is that there should be a fundamental distinction between basic research—learning how to do this [alter germline genes] in animal models and so forth—and the application of that research, which is where we obviously have to show a great deal more caution. What is absolutely fearful about a lot of the laws that came up in response to cloning is that they made no distinction. They went all the way back to the very core of this kind of research. Meetings like this are important because they help people gain an understanding about these distinctions and respond when laws are absolutely inappropriate.

One of the things that terrifies me about how laws get written is the realization that they're written by twenty-three-year-old staffers who are out to make a name, who studied this subject for three or four weeks. In general, those in Congress have even less idea of what this is all about, so it is a process that is not conducive to writing laws. But in spite of that, it ends up working surprisingly well.

Gregory Stock: Does anyone else have a comment to make about this subject? Lee?

Lee M. Silver: There is this false notion that species try to preserve their gene pools to try to preserve themselves. That is completely false. Species are always changing, and they even transform from one species to another. And as they change, their gene pools change naturally. This notion of a species trying to preserve itself is a false one right from the start.

Gregory Stock: Michael?

Controlling human evolution

Michael R. Rose: I would like to address the evolutionary issue. . . . Evolution is an incredibly complex process which is not suited to platitudes. Evolution can be spectacularly creative, so much so that many of the problems in artificial intelligence are now being solved using evolutionary algorithms. When design and optimality approaches fail now, artificial intelligence designers are using evolutionary techniques—basically, natural selection and genetic recombination—on computer programs. But just as you have to acknowledge the power and creativity of evolution, you also have to acknowledge its complete indifference to us as individuals. That's not what evolution is about at all. Evolution is about the transmission of DNA sequences down through time. We're just incidental things that get in the way. We're like the foot soldier in World War I, and we're sent out of the trenches into the enemy machine guns, and we die in our millions. And that's fine with evolution as long as our DNA gets into the next generation. This is, perhaps, part of my rebelliousness to the notion of "normal." I think what is normal is a catastrophic waste, and if one were simply to accept what evolution does as normal then, hell, you can give up on most everything that medicine does. You have to reject this concept of normal. You have to take what evolution does and look at it askance, exploit what it does well, and provide what it does not provide. And, of course, for those poor individuals who are afflicted by genetic diseases—which are the products of an evolutionary process in which mutation and selection together do not guarantee that everyone of us is genetically perfect, but only that most of us are genetically pretty good—their afflictions are a concrete example of where evolution has to be firmly rejected. The fact that, to evolution, we are disposable past a certain age is another candidate for rejecting what evolution normally does and doing something completely different. I think we need to seek an appropriate balance between respect for and use of what evolution does and rejection of what evolution does.

Gregory Stock: Along those same lines, I would like to express the notion that evolution, as it has operated in the past, has essentially stopped for the human species. Our future evolution will be intimately connected with the technologies that are being developed today. When you look forward, even a few centuries, it is difficult to imagine how you could separate any changes that occur to the human species from the technology that is evolving now and is now reflecting back upon ourselves. Does anyone have a comment to make about that general notion? John?

John Campbell: I suspect that the idea of us grabbing the reins of our own evolution is not new. Students of human evolution recognize that the major factor in the past history of humans—the past several million years in the development of humans—has been the tampering by humans with their own reproductive system, through sexual selection. Indeed, Darwin believed that sexual selection was the main factor that caused humans to evolve. He did not talk about the evolution of humans in his *Origin of the Species by Natural Selection.* He put it in a separate volume on natural selection in relation to sex and the origin of man. So, he put the origin of humans right in with sexual selection. L.S.B. Leakey thought the way to think about how we originated was that we autodomesticated ourselves. Other people have thought that the most important factor was the parent-offspring relationship, that the real selection pressure was the degree to which a mother protected her offspring. Undoubtedly, humans have been the main instruments in their evolution, the process which brought them to the status of being human. If we now start to tamper with our evolution, we are not doing something that is unique or unnatural or something that hasn't happened before. What I see as unique is that now we can bring our rationality to it, instead of having it based on sexual preference.

For the first time we understand that as a species we have the ability to self-evolve.

Gregory Stock: Dr. Koshland?

Daniel Koshland Jr.: We're doing evolution in test tubes now. In my laboratory we're using what's called combinatorial chemistry, which is what happens in evolution. You combine chemistry with the idea of selection in biology, and you make billions of mutants, of, say, little peptides. Then they are selected in your laboratory. Basically, that's what happens over evolutionary time in millions of years. This is now spreading throughout industry; the biotech industry, for instance, is using it to develop new drugs.

In some ways this comes back to germline engineering, because we've decided as a society that it's too cruel to get rid of less-effective or defective people, like those, for example, who have glasses. It really is crazy to discard a rational approach to helping our species, since we really have rejected the system that, as Dr. Campbell pointed out, has in a cruel way, over years and years, discarded the less fit. Now say we don't want to improve the species, because that would be too mean and inappropriate to the less able.

Gregory Stock: Dr. Hood, you would like to make a closing comment?

Leroy Hood: There is another way we can use evolution in absolutely incredible ways to help us decipher some of the most complicated of these "complex traits." One of the speakers mentioned—I think it was Lee Silver—that chimps and humans are 99 percent identical in their [DNA] sequences. One incredibly fascinating project would be to have a Chimp Genome Project and to compare the results with those from the Human Genome Project. The genes that would be enormously fascinating to compare are those that regulate the nervous system, for therein would be a great deal of the information that separates what we can do with our minds and learning and thinking from what a chimp can do. Also, you can use evolution in a lot of ways to gain fundamental insights into the kind of things we need to be able to manipulate in the future, if we want to fundamentally change schizophrenia, manic depression, and a lot of these very, very complex multifactorial diseases.

Gregory Stock: Does anyone else have a closing comment they feel burning within them?

Lee M. Silver: This is not something that is going to happen overnight or even within the next thirty or fifty or a hundred years. But for the first time we understand that as a species we have the ability to self-evolve. That's what the difference is with this new technology versus the sexual selection which occurred subconsciously in previous years. I mean, this is an incredible concept: that our species has the ability to self-evolve.

8
Triumph or Tragedy? The Moral Meaning of Genetic Technology

Leon R. Kass

Leon R. Kass is Addie Clark Harding professor at the University of Chicago. Trained in medicine and biochemistry, he writes frequently about bioethical issues such as human genetic engineering and physician-assisted suicide. With James Q. Wilson, he is coauthor of The Ethics of Human Cloning.

The public is right to doubt the ethics of applying gene-altering technology to humans. Unlike conventional medicine, this technology could affect not only existing individuals but others not yet born or even conceived. Knowledge of one's own genetic weaknesses may threaten human free will, and being able to change the genes of one's offspring may endanger human dignity by making children into manufactured commodities. Gene manipulation is likely to move from therapy (curing diseases) to enhancement, or adding characteristics that some members of society deem desirable. In doing so, it may alter the nature of the human species. It is thus a threat to humanity.

When, less than a half-century ago, James D. Watson and Francis Crick first revealed to the world the structure of DNA, no one imagined how rapidly genetic technology would develop. Within a few years, we shall see the completion of the Human Genome Project, disclosing the DNA sequences of all 100,000 human genes. [The project was completed in June 2000.] And even without complete genomic knowledge, biotech business is booming: according to a recent report by the research director for Smith Kline Beecham [a drug company], enough sequencing data are already available to keep his researchers busy for the next twenty years, developing early-detection screening techniques, rationally designed vaccines, genetically-engineered changes in malignant tumors leading to enhanced immune response, and, ultimately, precise gene therapy for specific diseases. In short, the age of genetic technology has arrived.

This technology comes into existence as part of the large humanitarian project to cure disease, prolong life, and alleviate suffering. As such, it occupies the moral high ground of compassionate healing. Who would not welcome surgery to correct the genetic defects that lead to sickle-cell anemia, Huntington's disease, and breast cancer, or to protect against the immune deficiency caused by the AIDS virus?

The scientists' attempt to cast the debate as a battle of beneficent and knowledgeable cleverness versus ignorant and superstitious anxiety should be resisted.

And yet genetic technology has also aroused considerable public concern. Even people duly impressed by the astonishing achievements of the last decades are nonetheless ambivalent about these new developments. For they sense that genetic technology, while in some respects continuous with the traditional medical project of compassionate healing, also represents something radically new and disquieting. For their own part, enthusiasts of this technology are often impatient with such disquiet, which they tend to attribute to scientific ignorance or else to outmoded moral and religious notions.

In my own view, the scientists' attempt to cast the debate as a battle of beneficent and knowledgeable cleverness versus ignorant and superstitious anxiety should be resisted. For the public is right to be ambivalent about genetic technology, and no amount of instruction in molecular biology and genetics should allay its—our—legitimate human concerns. In what follows, I mean to articulate some of those concerns, bearing in mind that genetic technology cannot be treated in isolation but must be seen in connection with other advances in reproductive and developmental biology, in neurobiology, and in the genetics of behavior—indeed, with all the techniques now and soon to be marshaled to intervene ever more directly and precisely into the bodies and minds of human beings. I shall proceed by raising a series of questions.

What is different about genetic technology?

At first glance, not much. Isolating a disease-inducing aberrant gene looks fairly continuous with isolating a disease-inducing intracellular virus; supplying diabetics with normal genes for producing insulin has the same medical goal as supplying them with insulin for injection.

Nevertheless, despite these obvious similarities, genetic technology is also decisively different. When fully developed, it will wield two powers not shared by ordinary medical practice. Medicine treats only existing individuals, and it treats them only remedially, seeking to correct deviations from a more or less stable norm of health. Genetic engineering, by contrast, will, first of all, deliberately make changes that are transmissible into succeeding generations and may even alter in advance specific future individuals through direct "germ-line" or embryo interventions. Secondly, genetic engineering may be able, through so-called genetic enhancement, to create new human capacities and hence new norms of health and fitness.

For the present, it is true, genetic technology is hailed primarily for its ability better to diagnose and treat disease in existing individuals. Confined to such practices, it would raise few questions (beyond the usual ones of safety and efficacy). Even intrauterine gene therapy for existing fetuses with diagnosable genetic disease could be seen as an extension of the growing field of fetal medicine. But there is no reason to believe that the use of gene-altering powers can be so confined, either in logic or in practice.

For one thing "germ-line" gene therapy and manipulation, affecting not merely the unborn but also the unconceived, is surely in our future. The practice has numerous justifications, beginning with the desire to reverse the unintended dysgenic effects of modern medical success. Thanks to medicine, for example, individuals who would have died from diabetes now live long enough to transmit their disease-producing genes. Why, it has been argued, should we not reverse these unfortunate changes by deliberate intervention? More generally, why should we not effect precise genetic alteration in disease-carrying sperm or eggs or early embryos, in order to prevent in advance the emergence of disease that otherwise will later require expensive and burdensome treatment? Why should not parents eager to avoid either the birth of afflicted children or the trauma of eugenic abortion be able to avail themselves of such alteration?

Genetic technology really is different. It can and will go to work directly and deliberately on our basic, heritable, life-shaping capacities, at their biological roots.

In sum, before we have had more than trivial experience with gene therapy for existing individuals—none of it thus far successful—sober people have called for overturning the current (self-imposed) taboo on germ-line modification. The line between these two practices cannot hold.

Despite the naive hopes of many, neither will we be able to defend the boundary between therapy and genetic enhancement. Will we reject novel additions to the human genome that enable us to produce, internally, vitamins or amino acids we now must get in our diet? Will we oppose the insertion of engineered foreign (or even animal) genes fatal to bacteria and parasites or offering us to increased resistance to cancer? Will we decline to make alterations in the immune system that will increase its efficacy or make it impervious to HIV? When genetic profiling becomes able to disclose the genetic contributions to height or memory or intelligence, will we deny prospective parents the right to enhance the potential of their children? Finally, should we discover—as no doubt we will—the genetic switches that control our biological clock, will we opt to keep our hands off the rate of aging or our natural human lifespan? Not a chance.

We thus face a paradox. On the one hand, genetic technology really is different. It can and will go to work directly and deliberately on our basic, heritable, life-shaping capacities, at their biological roots. It can take us beyond existing norms of health and healing—perhaps even alter fundamental features of human nature. On the other hand, precisely because the goals it will serve, at least to begin with, will be continuous with those of modern high-interventionist medicine, we will find its promise familiar and irresistible.

This paradox itself contributes to public disquiet: rightly perceiving a difference in genetic technology, we also sense that we are powerless to establish, on the basis of that difference, clear limits to its use. The genetic genie, first unbottled to treat disease, will go its own way, whether we like it or not.

How much genetic self-knowledge is good for us?

Quite apart from worries about genetic engineering, gaining genetic knowledge is itself a legitimate cause of anxiety, not least because of one of its most touted benefits—the genetic profiling of individuals.

The deepest problem connected with learning your own genetic sins and unhealthy predispositions is neither the threat to confidentiality and privacy nor the risk of discrimination in employment or insurance, important though these issues may be. It is, rather, the various hazards and deformations in living your life that will attach to knowing in advance your likely or possible medical future. To be sure, in some cases such foreknowledge will be welcome, if it can lead to easy measures to prevent or treat the impending disorder, and if the disorder in question does not powerfully affect self-image or self-command. But will and should we welcome knowledge that we carry a predisposition to Alzheimer's disease, schizophrenia, or some other personality or behavior disorder, or genes that will definitely produce at an unknown future time a serious but untreatable disease?

Still harder will it be for most people to live easily or wisely with less certain information—say, where multigenic traits are involved or where the predictions are purely statistical, with no clear implication for any particular "predisposed" individual. The recent case of a father who insisted that ovariectomy and mastectomy be performed on his ten-year-old daughter because she happened to carry the BRCA-1 gene for breast cancer shows dramatically the toxic effect of genetic knowledge.

Less dramatic but more profound is the threat to human freedom and spontaneity, a subject explored 25 years ago by the philosopher Hans Jonas. In a discussion of human cloning, Jonas argued eloquently for a "right to ignorance.":

> That there can be (and mostly is) too little knowledge has always been realized; that there can be too much of it stands suddenly before us in a blinding light. . . . The ethical command here entering the enlarged stage of our powers is: never to violate the right to that ignorance which is a condition for the possibility of authentic action; or: *to respect the right of each human life to find its own way and be a surprise to itself.* [Emphasis in the original]

To scientists convinced that their knowledge of predispositions can only lead to rational preventive medicine, Jonas's defense of ignorance will look like obscurantism. It is not. Although everyone remembers that Prometheus was the philanthropic god who gave to human beings fire and the arts, it is often forgotten that he also gave them the greater gift of "blind hopes," precisely because he knew that ignorance of one's own future fate was indispensable to aspiration and achievement. I suspect that many people, taking their bearings from life lived open-endedly rather than from preventive medicine practiced rationally, would prefer ignorance of the future to the scientific astrology of knowing their genetic profile. In a free society, that would be their right.

Or would it? This leads us to the next question.

What about freedom?

Even people who might otherwise welcome the growth of genetic knowledge and technology are worried about the coming power of geneticists, genetic engineers, and, in particular, governmental authorities armed with genetic technology.[1] Precisely because we have been taught by these very scientists that genes hold the secret of life, and that our genotype is our essence if not quite our destiny, we are made nervous by those whose expert knowledge and technique touch our very being. Even apart from any particular abuses or misuses of power, friends of human freedom have deep cause for concern.

The English humanist C.S. Lewis put the matter sharply in *The Abolition of Man* (1965):

> In reality, . . . if any one age really attains, by eugenics and scientific education, the power to make its descendants what it pleases, all men who live after it are the patients of that power. They are weaker, not stronger: for though we may have put wonderful machines in their hands we have preordained how they are to use them. . . . Man's conquest of Nature, if the dreams of some scientific planners are realized, means the rule of a few hundreds of men over billions upon billions of men. There neither is nor can be any simple increase of power on Man's side. Each new power won by man is a power over man as well. Each advance leaves him weaker as well as stronger. In every victory, besides being the general who triumphs, he is also the prisoner who follows the triumphal car.

Most genetic technologists will hardly recognize themselves in this portrait. Though they concede that abuses or misuses of power may occur, they see themselves not as predestinators but as facilitators, merely providing knowledge and technique that people can freely choose to use in making decisions about their health or reproductive choices. Genetic power, they will say, thus serves not to limit freedom but to increase it.

But as we can see from already existing practices like genetic screening and prenatal diagnosis, this claim is at best self-deceptive, at worst disingenuous [insincere]. The choice to develop and practice genetic screening and the choices of which genes to target for testing have been

---

1. It is remarkable that most discussions of genetic technology naively neglect its potential usefulness in creating biological weapons, such as, to begin with, antibiotic-resistant plague bacteria, or later, aerosols containing cancer-inducing or mind-scrambling viruses.

made not by the public but by scientists—and not on liberty-enhancing but on eugenic grounds. In many cases, practitioners of prenatal diagnosis refuse to do fetal genetic screening in the absence of a prior commitment from the pregnant woman to abort any afflicted fetus. In other situations, pregnant women who still wish not to know prenatal facts must withstand strong medical pressures for testing.

While a small portion of the population may be sufficiently educated to participate knowingly and freely in genetic decisions, most people are and will no doubt always be subject to the benevolent tyranny of expertise. Every expert knows how easy it is to get most people to choose one way rather than another simply by the way one raises the questions, describes the prognosis, and presents the options. The preferences of counselors will always overtly or subtly shape the choices of the counseled.

Economic pressures to contain health-care costs will almost certainly constrain free choice.

In addition, economic pressures to contain health-care costs will almost certainly constrain free choice. Refusal to provide insurance coverage for this or that genetic disease may eventually work to compel genetic abortion or intervention. State-mandated screening already occurs for PKU (phenylketonuria) and other diseases, and full-blown genetic-screening programs loom large on the horizon. Once these arrive, there will likely be an upsurge of economic pressures to limit reproductive freedom. All this will be done, of course, in the name of the well-being of children.

Already in 1971, the geneticist Bentley Glass, in his presidential address to the American Association for the Advancement of Science, enunciated "the right of every child to be born with a sound physical and mental constitution, based on a sound genotype." Looking ahead to the reproductive and genetic technologies that are today rapidly arriving, Glass proclaimed: "No parents will in that future time have a right to burden society with a malformed or a mentally incompetent child." It remains to be seen to what extent such prophecies will be realized. But they surely provide sufficient and reasonable grounds for being concerned about restrictions on human freedom, even in the absence of overt coercion, and even in liberal polities like our own.

What about human dignity?

Here, rather than in the more talked-about fears about freedom, lie our deepest concerns. Genetic technology, the practices it will engender, and above all the scientific teachings about human life on which it rests are not, as many would have it, morally and humanly neutral. Regardless of how they are practiced and taught, they are pregnant with their own moral meaning, and will necessarily bring with them changes in our practices, our institutions, our norms, our beliefs, and our self-conception. It is, I submit, these challenges to our dignity and humanity that are at the bottom of our anxiety over genetic science and technology. Let me touch briefly on four aspects of this most serious matter.

"Playing God." This complaint is too facilely dismissed by scientists and nonbelievers. The concern has meaning, God or no God. By it is meant one or more of the following: man, or some men, are becoming creators of life, and indeed of individual living human beings (in-vitro fertilization, cloning); not only are they creating life, but they stand in judgment of each being's worthiness to live or die (genetic screening and abortion)—not on moral grounds, as is said of God's judgment, but on somatic [bodily] and genetic ones; they also hold out the promise of salvation from our genetic sins and defects (gene therapy and genetic engineering).

Never mind the exaggeration that lurks in this conceit of man playing God: even at his most powerful, after all, man is capable only of playing God. Never mind the implicit innuendo that nobody has given to others this creative and judgmental authority, or the implicit retort that there is theological warrant for acting as God's co-creator in overcoming the ills and suffering of the world. Consider only that if scientists are seen in this godlike role of creator, judge, and savior, the rest of us must stand before them as supplicating, tainted creatures. That is worry enough.

Not long ago, at my own university, a physician making rounds with medical students stood over the bed of an intelligent, otherwise normal ten-year-old boy with spina bifida. "Were he to have been conceived today," the physician casually informed his entourage, "he would have been aborted." Determining who shall live and who shall die—on the basis of genetic merit—is a godlike power already wielded by genetic medicine. This power will only grow.

The road we are traveling leads all the way to the world of designer babies—reached not by dictatorial fiat but by the march of benevolent humanitarianism.

Manufacture and commodification. But, one might reply, genetic technology also holds out the promise of a cure for these life-crippling and life-forfeiting disorders. Very well. But in order truly to practice their salvific power, genetic technologists will have to increase greatly their manipulations and interventions, well beyond merely screening and weeding out. True, in some cases genetic testing and risk-management to prevent disease may actually reduce the need for high-tech interventions aimed at cure. But in many other cases, ever greater genetic scrutiny will lead necessarily to ever more extensive manipulation. And, to produce Bentley Glass's healthy and well-endowed babies, let alone babies with the benefits of genetic enhancement, a new scientific obstetrics will be necessary, one that will come very close to turning human procreation into manufacture.

This process has already crudely begun with in-vitro fertilization. It will soon take giant steps forward with the ability to screen in-vitro embryos before implantation; with cloning; and, eventually, with precise genetic engineering. The road we are traveling leads all the way to the world of designer babies—reached not by dictatorial fiat but by the march of benevolent humanitarianism, and cheered on by an ambivalent citizenry that also dreads becoming simply the last of man's manmade things.

Make no mistake: the price to be paid for producing optimum or even only genetically sound babies will be the transfer of procreation from the home to the laboratory. Increasing control over the product can only be purchased by the increasing depersonalization of the entire process and its coincident transformation into manufacture. Such an arrangement will be profoundly dehumanizing, no matter how genetically good or healthy the resultant children. And let us not forget the powerful economic interests that will surely operate in this area; with their advent, the commodification of nascent human life will be unstoppable.

Standards, norms, and goals. According to Genesis, God, in His creating, looked at His creatures and saw that they were good: intact, complete, well-working wholes, true to the spoken idea that guided their creation. What standards will guide the genetic engineers?

For the time being, one might answer, the norm of health. But even before the genetic enhancers join the party, the standard of health is being deconstructed. Are you healthy if, although you show no symptoms, you carry genes that will definitely produce Huntington's disease, or that predispose you to diabetes, breast cancer, or coronary artery disease? What if you carry, say, 40 percent of the genetic markers thought to be linked to the appearance of Alzheimer's? And what will "healthy" or "normal" mean when we discover your genetic propensities for alcoholism, drug abuse, pederasty, or violence? The idea of health progressively becomes at once both imperial and vague: medicalization of what have hitherto been mental or moral matters paradoxically brings with it the disappearance of any clear standard of health itself.

When genetic enhancement comes on the scene, standards of health, wholeness, or fitness will be needed more urgently than ever, but just then is when all pretense of standards will go out the window. "Enhancement" is a soft euphemism for "improvement," and the idea of improvement necessarily implies a good, a better, and perhaps even a best. If, however, we can no longer look to our previously unalterable human nature for a standard or norm of what is regarded as good or better, how will anyone know what constitutes an improvement? It will not do to assert that we can extrapolate from what we like about ourselves. Because memory is good, can we say how much more memory would be better? If sexual desire is good, how much more would be better? Life is good; but how much extension of life would be good for us? Only simplistic thinkers believe they can easily answer such questions.

Even the more modest biogenetic engineers, whether they know it or not, are in the immortality business.

More modest enhancers, like more modest genetic therapists and technologists, eschew grandiose goals. They are valetudinarians [people who worry about health], not eugenicists. They pursue not some faraway positive good but the positive elimination of evils: disease, pain, suffering, the likelihood of death. But let us not be deceived. Hidden in all this avoidance of evil is nothing less than the quasi-messianic goal of a painless, suffering-free, and finally immortal existence. Only the presence of such a goal justifies the sweeping-aside of any opposition to the relentless march of medical science. Only such a goal gives trumping moral power to the principle, "cure disease, relieve suffering."

"Cloning human beings is unethical and dehumanizing, you say? Never mind: it will help us treat infertility, avoid genetic disease, and provide perfect materials for organ replacement." Such, indeed, was the tenor of the June 1997 report of the National Bioethics Advisory Commission on Cloning Human Beings. Notwithstanding its call for a temporary ban on the practice, the only moral objection the commission could agree upon was that cloning "is not safe to use in humans at this time" because the technique has yet to be perfected. Even this elite ethical body, in other words, was unable to muster any other moral argument sufficient to cause us to forgo the possible health benefits of cloning.

The same argument will inevitably also justify creating and growing human embryos for experimentation, revising the definition of death to facilitate organ transplantation, growing human body parts in the peritoneal cavities of animals, perfusing newly dead bodies as factories for useful biological substances, or reprogramming the human body and mind with genetic or neurobiological engineering. Who can sustain an objection if these practices will help us live longer and with less overt suffering?

In order to justify ongoing research, these intellectuals were willing to shed not only traditional religious views but any view of human distinctiveness and special dignity, their own included.

It turns out that even the more modest biogenetic engineers, whether they know it or not, are in the immortality business, proceeding on the basis of a quasi-religious faith that all innovation is by definition progress, no matter what is sacrificed to attain it.

The tragedy of success. What the enthusiasts do not see is that their utopian project will not eliminate suffering but merely shift it around. We are already witnessing a certain measure of public discontent as a paradoxical result of rising expectations in the health-care field: although their actual health has improved, people's satisfaction with their current health status has remained the same or declined. But that is hardly the highest cost of medical success.

As Aldous Huxley made clear in his prophetic *Brave New World*, the conquest of disease, aggression, pain, anxiety, suffering, and grief unavoidably comes at the price of homogenization, mediocrity, pacification, trivialized attachments, debasement of taste, and souls without love or longing. Like Midas, bioengineered man will be cursed to acquire precisely what he wished for, only to discover—painfully and too late—that what he wished for is not exactly what he wanted. Or, worse than Midas, he may be so dehumanized he will not even recognize that in aspiring to be perfect, he is no longer even truly human.

The point here is not the rightness or wrongness of this or that imagined scenario—all this is admittedly highly speculative. I surely have no way of knowing whether my worst fears will be realized, but you surely have no way of knowing that they will not. The point is rather the plausibility, even the wisdom, of thinking about genetic technology, like the entire technological venture, under the ancient and profound idea of tragedy. In tragedy, the hero's failure is embedded in his very success, his defeats in his victories, his miseries in his glory. What I am suggesting is that the technological way of approaching both the world and human life, a way deeply rooted in the human soul and spurred on by the utopian promises of modern thought and its scientific crusaders, may very well turn out to be inevitable, heroic, and doomed.

To say that technology, left to itself as a way of life, is doomed, does not yet mean that modern life—our life—must be tragic. Everything depends on whether the technological disposition is allowed to proceed to its self-augmenting limits, or whether it can be restricted and brought under intellectual, spiritual, moral, and political rule. But here, I regret to say, the news so far is not encouraging. For the relevant intellectual, spiritual, and moral resources of our society, the legacy of civilizing traditions painfully acquired and long preserved, are taking a beating—not least because they are being called into question by the findings of modern science itself. The technologies present troublesome ethical dilemmas, but the underlying scientific notions call into question the very foundations of our ethics.

This challenge goes far beyond the notorious case of evolution versus biblical religion. Is there any elevated view of human life and human goodness that is proof against the belief, trumpeted by contemporary biology's most public and prophetic voices, that man is just a collection of molecules, an accident on the stage of evolution, a freakish speck of mind in a mindless universe, fundamentally no different from other living—or even nonliving—things? What chance have our treasured ideas of freedom and dignity against the teachings of biological determinism in behavior, the reductive notion of the "selfish gene" (or for that matter of "genes for altruism"), the belief that DNA is the essence of life, and the credo that the only natural concerns of living beings are survival and reproductive success?

Dangers to humanity

In 1997, the luminaries of the International Academy of Humanism—including the biologists Francis Crick, Richard Dawkins, and E.O. Wilson and the humanists Isaiah Berlin, W.V. Quine, and Kurt Vonnegut—issued a statement in defense of cloning research in higher mammals and human beings. Their reasons were revealing:

> What moral issues would human cloning raise? Some world religions teach that human beings are fundamentally different from other mammals—that humans have been imbued by a deity with immortal souls, giving them a value that cannot be compared to that of other living things. Human nature is held to be unique and sacred. Scientific advances which pose a perceived risk of altering this "nature" are angrily opposed. . . . As far as the scientific enterprise can de-

termine, [however] . . . [h]uman capabilities appear to differ in degree, not in kind, from those found among the higher animals. Humanity's rich repertoire of thoughts, feelings, aspirations, and hopes seems to arise from electrochemical brain processes, not from an immaterial soul that operates in ways no instrument can discover. . . . Views of human nature rooted in humanity's tribal past ought not to be our primary criterion for making moral decisions about cloning. . . . The potential benefits of cloning may be so immense that it would be a tragedy if ancient theological scruples should lead to a Luddite rejection of cloning.

In order to justify ongoing research, these intellectuals were willing to shed not only traditional religious views but any view of human distinctiveness and special dignity, their own included. They fail to see that the scientific view of man they celebrate does more than insult our vanity. It undermines our self-conception as free, thoughtful, responsible beings, worthy of respect because we alone among the animals have minds and hearts that aim far higher than the mere perpetuation of our genes. It undermines, as well, the beliefs that sustain our mores, institutions, and practices—including the practice of science itself. For why, on this radically reductive understanding of "the rich repertoire" of human thought, should anyone choose to accept as true the results of these men's "electrochemical brain processes," rather than his own? Thus do truth and error themselves, no less than freedom and dignity, become empty notions when the soul is reduced to chemicals.

There is, of course, nothing novel about reductionism, materialism, and determinism of the kind displayed here; they are doctrines with which Socrates contended long ago. What is new is that, as philosophies, they seem to be vindicated by scientific advance. Here, in consequence, is the most pernicious result of our technological progress—more dehumanizing than any actual manipulation or technique, present or future: the erosion, perhaps the final erosion, of the idea of man as noble, dignified, precious, or godlike, and its replacement with a view of man, no less than of nature, as mere raw material for manipulation and homogenization.

Hence our peculiar moral crisis: we adhere more and more to a view of human life that gives us enormous power and that, at the same time, denies every possibility of nonarbitrary standards for guiding the use of this power. Though well-equipped, we know not who we are or where we are going. We triumph over nature's unpredictabilities only to subject ourselves, tragically, to the still greater unpredictability of our capricious wills and our fickle opinions. That we do not recognize our predicament is itself a tribute to the depth of our infatuation with scientific progress and our naive faith in the sufficiency of our humanitarian impulses.

Does this mean that I am therefore in favor of ignorance, suffering, and death? Of killing the goose of genetic technology even before she lays her golden eggs? Surely not. But unless we mobilize the courage to look foursquare at the full human meaning of our new enterprise in biogenetic technology and engineering, we are doomed to become its creatures if not its slaves. Important though it is to set a moral boundary here, devise a regulation there, hoping to decrease the damage caused by this or that little rivulet, it is even more important to be sober about the true nature and meaning of the flood itself.

That our exuberant new biologists and their technological minions might be persuaded of this is, to say the least, highly unlikely. But it is not too late for the rest of us to become aware of the dangers—not just to privacy or insurability, but to our very humanity. So aware, we might be better able to defend the increasingly beleaguered vestiges and principles of our human dignity, even as we continue to reap the considerable benefits that genetic technology will inevitably provide.

9

Cloning Humans Is Ethical

Gregory E. Pence

Gregory E. Pence is professor of philosophy in the Schools of Medicine and Arts/Humanities at the University of Alabama, Birmingham. He teaches and writes extensively about biomedical ethics. His books in-clude Classic Cases in Medical Ethics.

Those who wish to propose moral rules governing human asexual re-production, or cloning, should ask themselves four questions: Does the rule intrude too much on personal liberty? What is the point of the moral rule? Why assume the worst motives? Why fear slippery slopes? The answers will reveal that, in most circumstances, cloning is ethical. It harms no one, violates only traditional moral rules that do not necessarily apply to today's society, would usually be done for good motives, and need not bring about disastrous changes.

The first stage [of modern moral philosophy] is one of grad-ual emergence from the traditional assumption that moral-ity must come from some authoritative source outside of human nature, into the belief that morality might arise from resources within human nature itself. It was a move-ment from the view that morality must be imposed on hu-man beings towards the belief that morality could be un-derstood as human self-governance or autonomy. This stage begins with the *Essays* of Michel de Montaigne and culmi-nates in the work of Kant, Reid, and Bentham.

During the second stage, moral philosophy was largely pre-occupied with the elaboration and defense of the view that we are individually self-governing, and with new objections and alternatives to it. The period extends from the assimila-tion of the works of Reid, Bentham, and Kant to the last third of the present century.

[In the last stage today], the attention of moral philosophers has begun to shift away from the problem of the autonomous individual toward new issues concerning public morality.

J.B. Schneewind, "Modern Moral Philosophy"[1]

Excerpted from *Who's Afraid of Human Cloning?* by Gregory E. Pence. Copyright © 1998 by Rowman & Littlefield Publishers, Inc. Reprinted with permission from Rowman & Littlefield Publishers, Inc.

In this essay, I describe four questions to ask when thinking about the morality of human asexual reproduction [cloning]. Before these descriptions, it will be helpful to have a case for focus. (This case, although realistic, does not refer to an actual case.)

The case of Sarah and Abe Shapiro

Sarah and Abe Shapiro yearned for a child for years before being able to have one. Both came from large Jewish families that put great emphasis on parental involvement with children and on family activities such as playing sports, eating nightly meals, and going on long camping trips.

Sarah and Abe also inherited something else from their families. Tay-Sachs disease runs in Jewish families of Eastern European origin. It is a lethal genetic disease that produces children who always die before they become teenagers.

Knowing their risk, Sarah and Abe used in vitro fertilization (IVF) so that any embryo implanted in Sarah could be screened for Tay-Sachs. In IVF, three embryos are often implanted in hopes that one will successfully gestate.

Such was the way Michael was created. Unfortunately, when the embryo that would become Michael was moving down Sarah's fallopian tube, it damaged her tube and rendered her infertile (her other tube was already damaged). So the Shapiros resigned themselves to having one child of their own and hoped, perhaps, to adopt another later.

When Michael was four, he and Abe were driving home from an outing when a drunk driver smashed into their car, instantly killing Abe and rendering Michael comatose, but with a beating heart sustained on a respirator.

After Abe's funeral, Sarah hoped for Michael to recover, praying to God for a miracle, which unfortunately did not come. During this time, she mourns the death of both Michael and Abe. After a year, her rabbi and therapist urged her "to move on with your life." They want her to agree to remove the respirator and allow Michael's body to die. She is only 40.

Sarah does not want to remarry. She is a writer and now owns her own home because of Abe's life insurance. However, she misses having a child in the house.

> *Especially in areas so personal as the make-up of the family and familial reproduction, the religious views of the majority have no place running federal policy.*

At this point, she decides to have one of her eggs removed, its nucleus taken out, and have the genes from Michael's body inserted in her egg to create a new embryo. After doing so, she will let Michael go. One of her reasons for using Michael's genes, she says, is that, "I couldn't bear to have a child who then died very young of Tay-Sachs." In this way, she knows her child will also be normal and be part of both her and Abe.

In many sessions, the rabbi, therapist, and infertility-physicians explore with Sarah the idea that she is merely attempting to replace Michael and that she has not fully accepted Michael's death. These professionals want to ensure that Sarah understands that the new child will be very different from Michael. They emphasize that Abe's influence will be missing, that Sarah's egg will contribute mitochondrial genes, that Sarah herself is now different, and so on.

Sarah claims that she is not trying to mechanically replace Michael and that she has accepted Michael's real death. She adds, "I know Michael and Abe are dead, but if God lets me bring forth this new child, whom I will call David, then Michael's and Abe's lives will not have been for nothing, for in David's life I can see, if not them, then at least their features and talents live on. Maybe I'll see Michael's way of laughing and Abe's swagger after he performs well in sports. What's wrong with that?"

A genetic counselor points out that she may also get the worst qualities from Abe and Michael, and is she prepared for that? "The worst qualities?" she ponders. "Well, they sure weren't perfect and they did have some of those, but I personally would rather have their worst qualities than just accept some anonymous sperm implanted in me, where the child will have no relation to Michael or Abe, and perhaps, to a history of Jews going back five thousand years."

Query 1—Does the rule intrude too much on personal liberty?

John Stuart Mill wrote *On Liberty* in 1859, and it contains an admirable distinction between private life and public morality, a distinction based on the concept of harm. Mill believed that a civilized society must promote certain ideals and discourage certain vices. Society can do this through its public policy while granting individuals a sphere of private action that is protected from interference by government. Power of the nation-state can be dangerous when used against the individual, and so the agents of government—such as police and military—should be forbidden to meddle in private life.

Equally, Mill held, the majority of citizens should be forbidden from becoming tyrannical. It should be forbidden from imposing its religious beliefs on a dissenting minority, even indirectly—say, by a judge who insists on a Christian prayer with a jury before they hear a case. It should be forbidden from censuring what is discussed publicly, say by a television station that decides that its viewers should not see homosexual characters. It is important to emphasize here that Mill believed that the majority's tyranny is normally done in the name of morality.

It is natural to ask where the line is to be drawn between private and public life. Mill's rough rule-of-thumb is called his *harm principle:* private life encompasses those actions of adults that are purely personal and put other people at no risk of harm. In such areas, there should be no interference by government—even for a person's own good. Consider nontraditional sex roles between two consenting adults (where the wife leaves home to work and the husband raises the children at home); even if other people consider these roles immoral, their relationship for Mill poses no moral question because no one else is affected.

Building on Mill's work, we can distinguish between four different areas where issues about human cloning arise: (1) personal life, (2) morality,

(3) public policy, and (4) the law. Issues of personal life are purely private and affect no one else. When someone else is affected, issues move from the personal to the realm of morality. When society attempts to promote certain positive values while at the same time tolerating personal disagreement with those values, we move into the third area, public policy.

Actions in the area of public policy, like those in the area of morality, do affect other people's interests, but persuasive actions in public policy are not necessarily condemned as immoral. Consider alcohol. Although society tries to discourage consumption of alcohol (by taxation) and regulates it (forbidding alcohol at elementary schools) people may drink in their homes without being viewed as immoral. Consider also adoption. Society wants adults to adopt needy children, and offers tax incentives to adults to so encourage this, but no one thinks it immoral for a childless couple not to adopt a baby.

This . . . fact—that motives and consequences determine the morality of an act—is a helpful one to keep in mind when we ask why a certain rule is still a good one.

These spheres overlap and shade into each other, and there is no exact criteria for separating one area from the next. The general goal is to limit the range of morality from two ends: first by carving out a zone of private, personal life, and second, by allowing society to encourage and discourage behaviors in public policy without explicit moral judgment or legal penalty. The general goal recognizes that we are all better off not moralizing every aspect of life.

One of the things Mill meant is that views that are essentially religious, even if held by the majority, should not be imposed on the minority. Especially in areas so personal as the make-up of the family and familial reproduction, the religious views of the majority have no place running federal policy.

Query 2—What is the point of the moral rule?

Instead of the usual question about ideal morality (about how morality ought to be), it is useful to consider how morality actually works. Call this the functional view of morality.

In this view, moral rules exist to adjudicate conflicts between the interests of persons. Because modern society contains many different kinds of people with many different points of view, moral rules are necessary for us to get along peacefully. In this functional view, the point of moral rules is not to prepare everyone for salvation or to create a purely religious state on earth. (These were the metaphysical beliefs associated with moral rules that at one time were quite functional.) Nor is the point of morality to create the greatest good for the greatest number of humans and animals on the planet. Nor is the point to create a perfectly rational, elegant theory of morality. Instead, the point is the more minimal one of getting along in a world where some resources will always be scarce, where interests of people conflict, and where people are interdependent and must cooperate.

So moral rules adjudicate social relations. Where they fail, the tougher ways of the law begin. Given that function, past moral rules may not always work in contemporary times, and when that happens, the nature of morality itself comes into question. For example, the very concept of having an interest has changed substantially over the last century, from covering one's household property to covering one's interest in pirated copies of one's book sold in China.

Moral rules in this functional sense are moot when there is no conflict, where the people have no real interests at stake, or where there are no existing people. For example, suppose Smith and I agree to share the planting of a boundary hedge along the property line on the west side of my yard, but my neighbor Jones on the eastern side is jealous of the cooperation between Smith and me, so much so that he objects to the joint project between Smith and me. Jones has no right to do so because he has no interests at stake. As so often happens in morality, his very objection creates a moral issue between Jones and me (because he is trying to interfere with my relations with my other neighbor) when there was no moral issue before.

Thus the point of moral rules is not to create an ideal society. Some philosophical vision of the future must do that, while moral rules allow us to get along enough to get there. In the technical language of moral philosophy, there is the theory of the right and the theory of the good. If we have the right theory of the right, we will allow different people to live their lives according to their view of the good.

Most popular discussions about cloning a human assume the worst possible motives in parents, but why on earth make such assumptions?

Application of this point to human asexual reproduction is obvious: if there is no conflict between two or more people, there is no moral issue present. Despite the widespread belief to the contrary, if no one is harmed by human asexual reproduction, then it raises no moral issue.

I want to also make a more general point here about the point of moral rules. The two great traditions that we have inherited from the past focus on two ways of evaluating moral acts: by their motives and by their consequences. Hence, if we want to know why an action is right, we can look at either the motives of the agents or the action's consequences. Judaeo-Christian ethics tends to focus on the motive of the act—what was in the agent's mind or heart—and not on what consequences occur. A secular ethics such as utilitarianism focuses on the actual consequences.

This surprisingly simple fact—that motives and consequences determine the morality of an act—is a helpful one to keep in mind when we ask why a certain rule is still a good one. Sometimes, a rule will become written in stone and we forget why it came about in the first place. If we carefully inspect the motives and consequences associated with that rule, we may sometimes discover that it is outdated.

Nor should we assume that the specific moral judgments that we make and that seem "obvious" to us will stand the test of time. As the Australian moral philosopher Peter Singer writes on this question:

> Why should we not rather make the opposite assumption, that all the particular moral judgments we intuitively make are likely to derive from discarded religious systems, from warped views of sex and bodily functions, or from customs necessary for the survival of the group in social and economic circumstances that now lie in the distant past? In which case, it would be best to forget all about our particular moral judgments, and start again from as near as we can get to self-evident moral axioms.[2]

For example, our culture traditionally has forbidden actively assisting a terminally ill person to die ("active euthanasia"), but it considers it permissible to merely watch such a person die slowly. So a basic rule in our culture is that allowing terminal patients to die is permissible, where assisting them is not.

This rule is outdated. How do we know? Because in both modes, the motives and consequences are the same. Situations often arise with terminal patients where the motives of everyone—including the patient himself—are to create a quick, painless death. Here the people intend quick death and quick death is the result. Given such a situation, it cannot matter morally whether the actions taken to hasten death are passive or active.[3]

Put differently, if the motives were bad and the consequences were bad, then the action would be bad according to either kind of moral theory. But it would make little sense to say that the description of the act as passive or as active really held the moral weight. To say so would be like saying that a performance of a piece of music was bad not because of how it was played but because of how it was classified.

Query 3—Why assume the worst motives?

The case of Sarah Shapiro is deliberately formulated to have a parent who has good motives about originating a child asexually. As the case shows, such a possibility is not unimaginable and, given the unpredictability of human life, a case such as this will one day arise.

Most popular discussions about cloning a human assume the worst possible motives in parents, but why on earth make such assumptions? Without evidence? If someone assumes that every person he meets is a secret racist or anti-Semite, we say he is paranoid, or a misanthrope, or warped. Why assume the worst motives when we are thinking about morality? Or in public policy? This way of thinking got us nowhere in the cold war, when the U.S. and Russia competed in the nuclear arms race and where it was assumed that Communists were evil people and Americans were saints. Why assume in public policy what we don't assume in ordinary life? We don't forsake participation in car pools that take our kids places because we fear that some parent may decide to kidnap the kids for ransom. Why should we assume worse when it comes to thinking about parents in public policy?

It has always been a trick of advocates of the status quo to assume the worst motives in humans. That is what the theory of original sin is all about. But humans are a lot better off today than a thousand years ago, and also a lot better off than a hundred years ago. And the main reason why is the electricity, antibiotics, clean water, efficient transportation, mass communication, and public education that humans have created. (Those who disagree know only the false, rose-colored versions of history seen in the mass media.) So why not trust humans rather than fear them? Who else has brought this progress? (If God has allowed humans to progress, why won't he allow them to progress more?)

An important corollary here is to ask about the evidence for assuming bad motives in ordinary people. If there is no such evidence, no such motives should be assumed. We have thousands of years of history with human parents and we know them well. We know that most parents most of the time do not have evil motives toward their children.

If we slipped down the slope, and many would deny we did, then at some point we took stock of where we were, changed our minds, and walked back up.

Nevertheless, many of our pundits assume the worst about us. Catholic University law professor Robert Destro wondered if cloned humans would have adequate legal rights "if they were created to perform specific work."[4] Why assume this? It is like saying that we should not admit emigrants to this country because they might by enslaved by natives. Why would a parent be so bigoted? ("Laura, dear, why don't we clone a little slave-child to walk the dog and clean the kitty litter?")

The Reverend Richard McCormick said that "the obvious motives for cloning a human were 'the very reasons you should not.'"[5] Obviously Father McCormick thinks it is "obvious" that couples have bad motives. He thinks that a couple might try to "create someone who could be a compatible organ donor." Really? Create your son and rip out his heart?

McCormick was probably thinking of the Ayala case where a couple conceived a daughter as a possible donor of bone marrow for their elder daughter dying of leukemia, and where they were lucky and had a new baby whose marrow matched.[6] But as medical sociologist Jay Hughes notes, there is all the difference in the world between renewable resources for transplantation, such as bone marrow, skin, urine, hair, and blood, and non-renewable human resources, such as hearts.[7]

Bioethicist Thomas Murray, a member of the Bioethics Advisory Commission, said, "Why are we uneasy about cloning? We might be worried over the dangers of excessive control over human reproduction, about the dangers of unbounded human pride."[8] But why assume that a government ban on human cloning is also not "excessive control over human reproduction?" Why assume that "unbounded human pride" is why couples would originate children by cloning? Why is giving couples more control over baby-making—which they have lacked through 99.9% of human history—a bad thing?

Why make such ridiculous assumptions about the motives of ordinary couples yet to have children? Go to your local neighborhood meeting,

Parents-Teacher Association night, or Kiwanis Club and ask yourself: are all those people the kind of people who have bad motives? To assume bad motives in a crack addict or an alcoholic parent is understandable because we know that their free will has been largely overtaken by a drug. The drug will win out over any motive for a child's welfare. But most parents are not drug-dependent, nor are they malignant narcissists. Indeed, when we are almost exclusively discussing parents who want and plan for a child, and have good resources to raise such a child, we have adverse selection into that subset of parents who are unlikely to have such bad motives.

Query 4—Why fear slippery slopes?

One of the central objections to cloning a human concerns the idea of a slippery slope, perhaps the second most famous idea in ethics (behind the Golden Rule). True, it will be allowed, extraordinary circumstances may make it plausible in the Shapiro case to think about allowing human asexual reproduction, but if that case is allowed, then another similar case must be allowed, until we get to some really terrible scenarios.

For example, twenty years ago in the debate about in vitro fertilization, Leon Kass objected that:

> At least one good humanitarian reason can be found to jus-
> tify each step. The first step serves as a precedent for the sec-
> ond and the second for the third, not just technologically
> but also in moral argument. Perhaps a wise society would
> say to infertile couples: "We understand your sorrow, but it
> might be better not to go ahead and do this."[9]

The rough idea here is that if a small, benign change is allowed, it will inevitably lead to another, less benign change, and so on through a series of inevitable steps, until a point is reached where a very bad outcome is at hand. A corollary is that, once the first change is accepted, there is no easy way to stop until the last, bad point is reached. Hence, the inference is made, better not to change at all.

The slippery slope is, for better or worse, also a central idea in bioethics. Because bioethics has been at the forefront of change over the last decades, "slope predictions" have been common. Indeed, every time real social change occurs, it scares most people, and some moralists will predict that the sky will soon fall: "The dawn of the era of cloning is a lit-tle like splitting the atom," said Dr. Glenn Bucher, president of the Grad-uate Theological Union in Berkeley, California, "with enormous prospects for evil and enormous prospects for good."[10]

But we must not be manipulated by predictions made at the drop of a hat. In the one above, with what is Bucher comparing "enormous prospects for evil?" The Holocaust? The Mongol invasion of Europe? AIDS? Does he really mean to indirectly refer to the atomic bomb?

One famous book was full of slope predictions. Thirty years ago, Alvin Toffler breathlessly coined the term "future shock" to "describe the shattering stress and disorientation that we induce in individuals by sub-jecting them to too much change in too short a time."[11] His *Future Shock* sold millions of copies and he was anointed as the futurologist whose om-niscience revealed the (mostly dire) future of humanity. Toffler hyperventilated that social change was occurring so fast that we were losing all our moorings and would soon be adrift in a sea of social chaos. (Alasdair McIntyre's books push the same theme at the theoretical level in ethics.[12])

Toffler wrote *Future Shock* between the years of 1965 and 1970, when the industrialized, Western world was rapidly changing. Those years witnessed big changes in music, sex roles, blended families, suspicion of authority and old age, and a new tolerance for drugs, sexual experimentation, contraception, abortion, and divorce.

What Toffler failed to predict was that too much change creates an opposing reaction toward stability. By 1981, when AIDS began, the conservative reaction was already well under way and it kept rolling through the 1990s: couples reverted to traditional sex roles, nuclear families were again seen as an ideal, hostility renewed towards illegal drugs (especially cocaine and heroin), realization occurred that contraception and abortion weren't stopping teenage pregnancy, and divorce was seen to hurt children and hence, to be too easy. If we slipped down the slope, and many would deny we did, then at some point we took stock of where we were, changed our minds, and walked back up.

The specific predictions made by *Future Shock* about human cloning, artificial wombs, and genetic engineering are lessons in caution. Nobel Laureate geneticist Joshua Lederberg predicted to Toffler—sometime between 1965 and 1970—that "somebody may be doing it [cloning] right now with mammals. It wouldn't surprise me if it comes out any day now."[13] As for cloning humans, Lederberg gave it (at most) fifteen years. Lederberg also thought that the time was "very near" when "the size of the brain . . . would be brought under direct developmental control," when we could create much bigger, better brains for children.

Be wary of slope predictions and don't let them make you fear the changes that may bring you a better future.

One of the great problems for a non-scientist in the field is to evaluate the ability of someone like Lederberg to make such predictions outside his real field of expertise. Lederberg sounded perspicacious at the time, and certainly exciting (and Toffler was certainly selling excitement about the future in his book), but Lederberg ignored countless barriers, such as the ability of the government—if it chose—to ban funding for such research.

And as for Toffler, of course it is the tone that sells a book, especially a tone of impending Armageddon:

> It is important for laymen to understand that Lederberg is by no means a lone worrier in the scientific community. His fears about the biological revolution are shared by many of his scientific colleagues. The ethical, moral, and political questions raised by the new biology simply boggle the mind. Who shall live and who shall die? What is man? Who shall control research into these fields? How shall new find-

ings be applied? Might we not unleash horrors for which man is totally unprepared? In the opinion of many of the world's leading scientists the clock is ticking for a "biological Hiroshima."[14]

Well, not really. And I would like to see the hard data that proved, even then, that "many" of the world's top scientists feared such a future, or that Lederberg's views were not confined to a small, speculative minority. In fact, Lederberg was very alone in going out on a limb with his highly speculative predictions.

In the next paragraph, Toffler quotes E. Hafez (a man who, he tells us, is an "internationally respected biologist") who predicted in 1965 that,

> . . . within a mere ten to fifteen years, a woman will be able to buy a tiny embryo, take it to her doctor, have it implanted in her uterus, carry it for nine months and then give birth to it as though it had been conceived in her own body.

It wasn't until 1978 that Louise Brown was born by in vitro fertilization and the first American IVF baby didn't come until 1980. Only in 1996 did some desperate, infertile couples start to pay young women for eggs that would be fertilized with the husband's sperm for implantation in the older woman. Couples still can't "buy" an embryo.

Toffler next quoted Daniele Petrucci (by the way, all his quotes from Hafez and Petrucci came from a sensationalistic article in *Life* magazine in 1965, so Toffler was taking *Life*'s word about the credentials of these men and women, who claimed that artificial wombs are just around the corner):

> Indeed, it will be possible at some point to do away with the female uterus altogether. Babies will be conceived, nurtured and raised to maturity outside the human body. It is clearly only a matter of years before the work begun by Dr. Daniele Petrucci in Bologna . . . makes it possible for women to have babies without the discomfort of pregnancy.[15]

Petrucci had claimed to have fertilized a human egg in vitro, grown it for 29 days, and then destroyed it because it was growing as a monster. What Toffler didn't discover then was that the evidence for this claim was never provided by Petrucci and the claim was later dismissed as fraudulent. (This fraud was harmful because it fueled later worries that IVF might produce monstrous babies—a fear also raised about cloning.) And of course, we are nowhere near having a real artificial womb.

In (what we can now see as) a hilarious scenario, Toffler somberly quotes Hafez's suggestion that,

> fertilized eggs might be useful in the colonization of planets. Instead of shipping adults to Mars, we could ship a shoebox full of such cells and grow them into an entire city size population of humans. Dr. Hafez observes, ". . . why send full-grown men and women aboard space ships? Instead, why not ship tiny embryos, in the care of a competent biologist . . . We miniaturize other spacecraft components. Why not the passengers?"[16]

Of course, Toffler could not resist the standard, dire predictions about eugenics, about a super race, and about state-controlled genetic enhancement. He eagerly quotes a kooky Soviet biologist predicting a "genetic arms race" between the Cold War enemies. For Toffler, "we are hurtling toward the time when we are able to breed both super- and sub-races. . . . We will be able to create super-athletes, girls with super-mammaries. . . ."

All these predictions were presented not as science fiction but as factual predictions. Toffler certainly got a lot of attention, but is his legacy a good one? On the good side, he scared people, and made them realize a lot of change had occurred in a few years. On the other side, he also made people feel that the change was uncontrollable and that we could never go back. In those aspects, his legacy has not been a good one.

Other breathlessly made predictions haven't come true. In the 1960s, computers were seen as the oppressive agents of the State, but in fact personal computers later created new ways of sharing ideas that helped bring down Communism all over the world. Physician-assisted dying for competent, terminal adults in Holland was predicted to turn that peaceful country into an ethical hell, but the practice has been going on for twenty-five years with hardly any bad results. Abortion has been legal in America for a similar twenty-five years and American society continues to function quite nicely.

All these changes—with computers, assisted reproduction, euthanasia, and abortion—were predicted by various seers to land us on an inexorable slide down the slippery slope. None of them came true. So the lesson here is easy: be wary of slope predictions and don't let them make you fear the changes that may bring you a better future.

Finally, one way that the first and last tests of this chapter are linked is that the slippery slope predictions often assume bad motives in parents. Ostensibly, desires to have children who lack genetic dysfunction and to make one's children as talented, healthy, and lovable as possible, do not seem like the pit at the bottom of a slippery slope—although from the way many pundits talk about the slippery slope, one might think it so.

I have offered four questions to ask when we discuss the ethics of human asexual reproduction. Of course, these tests are applicable to many other issues in ethics. In thinking about originating humans by cloning, we should not think of such origination as being a moral issue unless someone is harmed, not assume that traditional moral rules are always right because the problems they address may change, not assume the worst motives in parents, and not let predictions about slippery slopes make us fear change.

Notes

1. J.B. Schneewind, "Modern Moral Philosophy," in Peter Singer (ed.), *A Companion to Ethics* (Cambridge, Mass.: Blackwell, 1991), 147.

2. Quoted by James Rachels, in his *Can Ethics Provide Answers? And Other Essays in Moral Philosophy* (Lanham, Md.: Rowman & Littlefield, 1997), 8; from Peter Singer, "Sidgwick and Reflective Equilibrium," *Monist* 58 (1974): 516.

3. See James Rachels, "Active and Passive Euthanasia," *New England Journal of Medicine* 292 (9 January 1975), 78–80.

4. Gustav Niebuhr, "Cloned Sheep Stirs Debate on Its Use on Humans," *New York Times,* 1 March 1997.

5. Gustav Niebuhr, "Cloned Sheep. . . ."

6. See Gregory Pence, *Classic Cases in Medical Ethics*, 2nd ed. (New York: McGraw-Hill, 1995), 296.

7. Jay Hughes, Medical College of Wisconsin Medical Ethics listserv discussion, September 4, 1995. Transplanting a lobe of a liver or lung, or one kidney where two are functioning, is not transplanting a renewable resource but it is also not like transplanting a heart, which can only be done if a person is dead while his heart continues to beat.

8. "Overview on Cloning," *Los Angeles Times,* 27 April 1997.

9. *Newsweek,* 7 August, 1978, 71.

10. Gustav Niebuhr, "Cloned Sheep. . . ."

11. Alvin Toffler coined the term in 1965 in an article in *Horizon* magazine. The quotation is from his later book, *Future Shock* (New York: Bantam Books, 1970), 2.

12. Alasdair McIntyre, *After Virtue* (South Bend, Ind.: Indiana University Press, 1981.)

13. Alvin Toffler, *Future Shock,* 198.

14. Alvin Toffler, *Future Shock,* 198.

15. Alvin Toffler, *Future Shock,* 199–200.

16. Alvin Toffler, *Future Shock,* 200.

10

Cloning Humans
Is Not Ethical

Jorge L.A. Garcia

*Jorge L.A. Garcia is a professor of philosophy at Rutgers University. He
has also been a Fellow in Ethics at Harvard University and a senior research scholar at the Kennedy Institute of Ethics. He has written many
books and articles on theoretical and practical ethics, including* "It Just
Ain't Fair": The Ethics of Health Care for African-Americans.

Cloning of humans can never be ethical. It muddies the concepts
of family and parenthood, adding to the strain of modern family
life. It degrades the dignity of the person cloned by making him
or her subhuman, a manufactured product. It could lead to changing the human species and rejecting all children that do not measure up to parents' standards. The positive features of helping infertile or homosexual couples bear children are not important
enough to make cloning acceptable on the grounds of justice.
Cloning attacks human life by treating it as if it were of merely instrumental value, to be bestowed at will.

In one of Hegel's rare memorable passages, he remarks that the Owl of
Minerva takes flight to paint its gray on gray at the end of day. He seems
to have meant two things: that philosophy does little more than give intellectual expression to the spirit of the times and that it does even that
rather late, as the *Zeitgeist* [spirit of the times] is itself changing. Whatever
their truth as general claims about philosophy, they certainly capture the
discipline of bioethics. Practices that once outraged the common sensibility are now all the rage. Bioethicists, true to Hegel's vision, have entered the stage wringing their hands over some new practice, but quickly
changed their tune as social attitudes changed from hesitation and dis-
approval to cheery contentment. Indeed, as the first wave of medically
and theologically trained writers on medical ethics has been replaced by
today's crop of lawyers, policy specialists, analytic philosophers, and
those who revel in the neologism *ethicists*, they have become so adept at
this that they have gotten ahead of the curve of attitudinal shift. That is

not to say that they actually cause change, but they have removed an important cautionary voice, a brake against brash and sweeping transformations. In the past, intellectuals played an important cultural role in cautioning against haste, calling for reflection, reminding of past troubles, articulating traditional cultural commitments and a sense of continuity with forebears, and so on. In contrast, today's secularized clerisy of ethics intellectuals are among the most vocal in assuaging any lingering moral doubts about the new agenda pushed by researchers and the increasingly consumer-driven, market-modeled medical industries. A December 1997 *New York Times* headline caught this phenomenon nicely in the area that concerns us here: "On Cloning Humans, 'Never' Turns Swiftly into 'Why Not'?" The story notes that after the initial near-unanimous outcry against cloning humans that immediately followed the announcement of the Dolly experiment's success, "scientists have become sanguine about the notion of . . . cloning a human being."[1] Bioethicists' uncharacteristically negative initial reaction to the renewed talk of cloning humans is, in 1998, a cause of some embarrassment and, barely a year since Dr. Wilmut's announcement and less than a year after the National Bioethics Advisory Commission (NBAC) report, we were already in the midst of a full-scale moral reconsideration.

This is not a bad thing. Medical ethics probably suffers from too little reconsideration, not too much. Indeed, I think that one of the problems in some of the new literature on cloning is precisely that it treats as definitively settled moral questions about the status of the embryo and so-called preembryo, the moral legitimacy of abortion and in vitro fertilization done for more or less any reason, and other matters where some consensus may or may not be emerging among secular elites, but where nothing has really been proven morally, even if there is such a thing as moral proof. There is no reason, then, to decry the raising of the question the *Times* article heralds: Why not? However, the question should not be treated as an impatient challenge to put up or shut up, lest some new medical agendum be delayed. The philosophical approach is to treat the question as an inquiry into the reasons for which human cloning might be morally objectionable.[2] This is the spirit in which I will treat it here. Where the *Times* article notes a shift in attitudes from "never" to "why not"? the attitudes behind the two utterances are not opposed in principle. We can deny that cloning people is ever morally permissible and also inquire into what makes that true. Hence my subtitle, "Never *and* Why Not."

A bioethicist's view of human cloning

Gregory Pence's *Who's Afraid of Human Cloning?* (1998) is one of the first book-length treatments by a philosophically trained bioethicist since the announcement of the Dolly experiment's success, which defends human cloning as ethical. For that reason, and the fact that it is being marketed to a mass audience as a general-interest paperback on current affairs and science, it warrants attention.

You might have thought that even if the initial reaction against human cloning was inadequately thought through, there are serious problems about the practice. Yet as Pence makes clear in his very title, this is not his view. Hesitation about its licitness is just a matter of fear, not rea-

son. He warns us against "fear of a change, fear of changing human nature, fear of humans having more choice and control." This is just a strug-
gle between the "fatalistic view . . . that everything is changing too fast"
and those who distrust people, on one side, and "voluntarists," those who
believe "we have the wisdom to use new knowledge to help people" and
are "more optimistic," on the other.[3] Pence continues, "There is nothing
about change itself," we discover, "that is bad." With this hard-won in-
sight, he thinks, we can "take a more assertive stance toward the future of
humanity."[4] One might think that the end of humanity's most destructive
and barbarous century calls for more caution than Pence's none-too-
searching question, "So why not trust humans rather than fear them?"[5]
Reflect for a moment on what Arendt called "the banality of evil." Recall
what nice, ordinary people did or let happen in Germany, or Alabama, or
Siberia, or Soweto, or Tibet, in just the last few generations. Then follow
the procedure Pence recommends in considering whether we might use
the new technologies in ways that harm people: "Go to your local neighborhood meeting, Parents-Teacher Association night, or Kiwanis Club and
ask yourself: are all those people the kind who have bad motives?"[6] Those
with sufficient self-knowledge may not reach the answer Pence wants.

---

*Practices that once outraged the common sensibility
are now all the rage.*

People always worry about new medical practices, Pence thinks, and
the facts prove them wrong. After all, he says, "Physician-assisted dying
for competent, terminal adults in Holland was predicted to turn that
peaceful country into an ethical hell, but the practice has been going on
twenty-five years with hardly any bad results."[7] Justice Souter, whose con-
curring opinion in the 1997 assisted-suicide cases legal commentators saw
as almost inviting opportunity to find a more limited constitutionally
protected right, seems to have held back in these cases largely because of
the widespread abuses of the rules putatively governing physician-
assisted suicide in the Netherlands.[8] Does not involuntary euthanasia, un-
reported and unpunished, count as a bad result?

Despite those concerned about dangers of widespread human
cloning, we are not to worry: "For every high-minded couple who produced a superior child by NST [nuclear somatic transfer, a type of human
cloning] there would be a Brazilian couple who produced nine children
by normal sex."[9] Even within the often openly eugenicist discourse of
many proponents of human cloning, this explicit contrast of the high-
minded and superior on the one side and the Brazilian on the other is
shocking. But it is presumably acceptable to speak of Latin American reproductive customs with open contempt because these people are likely
to be Christians, especially Catholics or evangelicals. Those who are concerned about abortion and respect for human embryos are considered
foolish extremists. Richard Lewontin has questioned the conspicuous absence of testimony before the president's commission from Christian fun-
damentalists.[10] For Pence, however, too much was heard even from main-
line Protestant and Jewish thought, too much from religious people. Even

government regulation of cloning and other techniques of artificial reproduction is to be avoided because government is too easily pressured by "extreme religious groups."[11] He does not seem to have in mind those whose views, like those of his intellectual hero, Joseph Fletcher, are extreme in their enthusiasm for new manipulations of and interventions in the beginning and end of life.

Those who are concerned about abortion and respect for human embryos are considered foolish extremists.

Lutheran theologian Gilbert Meilander worries that cloning might not comport with Genesis's picture of human beings divinely enjoined to sustain human life through procreation. According to Pence, "The problem with Protestants justifying their views on biblical passages is that they only go there to justify what they already believe, not to find guidance."[12] It seems rather harsh to accuse a believer of abusing his or her own scriptures, seeking in them not the word of the God he or she thinks therein revealed but only endorsement of existing prejudices. No fair-minded person would make such a charge against a person, let alone a whole sect, without first entertaining the possibility that the thinker might indeed have sought and received guidance from the passage, might indeed have read and reflected on it many times. Meilander holds that a child is a gift from God and that we should strive so to see it, a striving he thinks cloning repudiates and makes more difficult.

Pence is in a hurry and Meilander's "gift" talk threatens to slow things down. All this fretting about God and ethics is "holding hostage important medical research," after all.[13] That Pence cannot abide. "When are we allowed to choose to have better babies?" he asks. "Never? When are we allowed to say to the Giver of the gift, 'Gee, couldn't you do any better than that?'"[14] "Better babies," "superior children" for the "high-minded" through cloning? Or Latinos rutting away—beneath garish images of Jesus on the bedroom wall, no doubt—turning out their litters of human inferiors? The contrast latent in Pence's imagery is now manifest. We should turn to his more thematic discussion of the moral case against cloning. However, before we get to that, we must pause to clear up some confusions Pence introduces about moral reasoning.

Ethical thinking

I have said that my interest here is to affirm the view that human cloning is not permissible morally (my "never") and to begin exploring some reasons for which it is not (my "why not"). If it is wrong, it is wrong for reasons. Notice, however, that this does not entail that in order for someone to know (or justifiably to believe) that it is wrong, he or she must first know why it is. It is an ontological point that has nothing to do with moral epistemology. Pence claims, for example, that "philosophers and bioethicists are very suspicious about 'knowing what you want to do' [in condemning something morally], but not knowing 'why' it is morally wrong." And plainly, he thinks their suspicions are right. In his view, "if the balance of reasons favors one side over another, we know that the right side is the one with the better reasons."[15] This may be right, but it is unwarranted. The reason for my doubt is precisely that this view does not seem to permit us to say that a position may be right but is unwarranted for us to assert at a certain time.

This principle would be nonsense as a general epistemological claim. If I claimed never to know what color or figural qualities a thing had until I knew why it had them, I would merely be deceiving myself. What is supposed to make the moral case so radically different? As in many other matters, we come to moral knowledge through various combinations of perception, testimony, inference, reflection, analysis, and empirical investigation. Of course, when I know that something is wrong, I often (but need not) also know some respect in which it is wrong. Still, it hardly follows that the "balance of reasons" must always favor the position that is, in fact, correct. Certainly, it need not if the reasons intended are merely the ones so far presented at a certain point in the discussion. Nor need the correct side even be favored by the balance of reasons available for our inspection. Maybe we just do not know yet what makes the thing wrong, as we do not know what grounds or causes many of its other qualities. Of course, there are forms of antirealism according to which saying something is wrong is just saying how the discussion of it is proceeding. And there are forms of constructivism according to which what is wrong is made wrong by a process of moral deliberation. I doubt any such metaethical theory is correct, but even if one proves true, that hardly warrants confidence that the correct moral position is always the one supported by the balance of reasons. So, as in other areas of inquiry, even if the moral arguments against human cloning were unpersuasive, weaker than those on the other side, that would not entail that the "right" view is that cloning is not wrong.

When I know that something is wrong, I often (but need not) also know some respect in which it is wrong.

This recalls Peter Singer's skeptical approach to so-called moral intuitions. Singer asks why we should not distrust our intuitive moral judgments about particular cases as "derive[d] from discarded religious systems, from warped views of sex and bodily functions, or from customs necessary for the survival of the group in social and economic circumstances that now lie in the distant past? In which case," he continues, "it would be best to forget all about our particular moral judgments, and start again from as near as we can get to self-evident moral axioms."[16]

I cannot pursue the issue of moral epistemology here. Permit me just to observe that what is required is to show that the discarded religious systems are false; that, whatever their truth or falsity, these systems' moral views did not capture important truths about human beings and their needs, service to which may explain the endurance of those moral intuitions; that warped views of sex are more likely to be found in traditional views than in more modern ones; and that we are likely to come closer to self-evidence at the level of general principles than we are at the level of judgments about particular forms of behavior, such as human cloning. Indeed, Mill himself conceded that we are more certain about particular judgments we make about this lie or that assault than we are about such generalizations as the utilitarians' own happiness principle.[17] My own view is that the lesson to be learned from thinking about intuitions—general and particular, old and new—is that we should be distrustful of the least reliable of intuitive judgments, that is, those that have arisen recently to allow us to feel all right about ourselves as we engage in practices long recognized as perverse. However, that does much to undercut a line of reasoning popular among the fans of human cloning and other new medical practices. For example, they argue that cloning for sex selection, to tailor children to parents' (or others') design specifications, or as a source of tissue donations is not wrong because something similar is sometimes done using in vitro fertilization (IVF), where (they say) it does not elicit the horror it used to.[18] That frequency has eroded the sense of moral horror some people feel over such practices does not mean that they now pass some test of acceptability before respectable intuitions. I should say the same about the view that we have somehow generally come to know that human life does not exist in utero or, if it does, that it deserves no protection there—that we have a right to decide exactly how and when to die. (What of the man who chooses to go out in mid-orgy with the Spice Girls in the Super Bowl half-time show?) Where is our distrust of received moral opinion when we need it?

There is ground for concern that, at a time when it is conceded all around that family life is strained, . . . cloning muddies the concepts of family and parenthood.

Returning to Pence, let us examine another claim about moral thinking and theory. He claims that Mill's famous harm principle, which holds that state prohibitions on liberty are permissible only when the prohibited behavior harms someone, "does not merely champion an area of personal life free from governmental interference, but also an area free from moral criticism."[19] It is difficult to see how this could be right as an interpretation of Mill's principle, but what is more important is that it is difficult to see how it could be a correct moral principle.[20] If a range of my actions is free from *all* moral criticism, even my own, then how can I undertake moral reform by acknowledging my own past wrongdoing in that area and seeking to avoid such behavior in the future? Is that area of my conduct to be free only from other people's moral criticism? Then what room would there be for me to seek your moral guidance in a matter of my private life? Even if the state should not intervene, can it really be correct that there is nothing morally objectionable in my conducting my private affairs from racial or ethnic or gender or religious prejudice? Or is it that such conduct is wrong, but that nobody has any business telling me so? If so, then how do I learn to reform morally? And what becomes of freedom of speech in this new gag-ruled version of "liberalism?"

At this point, I turn to consider some of the principal moral objections raised against human cloning. My aim in the next section is not to develop any of these arguments into decisive proofs of the immorality of human cloning but merely to point out difficulties in some efforts to counter them.

Some reasons against human cloning

Certainly, there is good reason to find the prospect of human cloning troubling. It appears in several ways to endanger society and those involved as donors or in gestation. It plainly poses a threat to the dignity and equality of women when, by plan, their childbearing loses its normal and proper origin in an act of spousal love. Pence realizes this possibility but poses no serious response. Instead, at this point he invokes his unusual interpretation of Mill's harm principle. Beyond that, he simply affirms that "women fearing increased sexism from the introduction of NST have a knock-down argument to any sexist fantasy about reproducti[ve exploitation] . . . they can simply refuse to get pregnant, refuse to stay pregnant, or refuse to gestate a fetus any more."[21] This comment misses the point of the objection several times over. The point is not about the consequences of desexed reproduction (i.e., whether it will increase sexism). Rather, it is about whether reproduction by human cloning already treats the gestating mother in a demeaning way.[22] In any case, it is no response to this concern to say that women can escape the degradation. For one thing, such ways out as sacrificing her child before its birth are already tragic. For another, a degradation eventually escaped is still a degradation and therefore something that should not be tolerated in the first place.

Similarly, there is good reason to worry that human cloning as it becomes widespread even as an available option depreciates and denatures both sexual relations and reproduction by making the former merely one alternative among many for the latter. Consider the view of the sexual that Alan Goldman calls "plain sex." This view understands sexual activity in terms of sexual desire, itself conceived simply as desire for tactile bodily contact and its pleasures.[23] It clearly fails to capture the sexual. It does not even successfully differentiate sexual activity from a vengeful desire to poke somebody. Understanding sex in terms of sexual desire gets things backwards. It completely misses the sexual because the very term and its cognates enter our vocabulary in differentiating groups, organs, and activities defined by their role in a certain mode of reproduction. Not all sex does or should result in reproduction, of course, but the idea that we can conceptualize the realm of the sexual without mention of reproduction is one of those ideas it seems only a modern intellectual could have.[24] Others would know better.

Again, there is ground for concern that, at a time when it is conceded all around that family life is strained, difficult, and damaging especially to children, cloning muddies the concepts of family and parenthood. This is especially likely in some of the bizarre scenarios where, for example, a mother bears the clone of her own grandfather or herself. Lewontin claims each clone will have two parents, just like everyone else, apparently meaning the male and female whose chromosomes joined to shape the principal gene donor's genome.[25] Another writer suggests that "a clone may have four 'genetic' parents" plus two (or more) additional mothers.[26] What matters is that the mother may bear (and thus be gestational mother of) someone whose genetic parents (in Lewontin's sense of "parent") are her own great-grandparents. In another, she is gestational mother of someone whose genetic parents are her own. In still other scenarios, identical twins are born years, even decades, apart. What sense can we make of generations in such a family? Indeed, in what sense is it family when the relationships that constitute it no longer match those constitutive of family life? Some people are sanguine that the family can easily be "reconceived" or "revisioned." More sober minds will want to proceed with caution here with what Aristotle considered the fundamental unit of society. It is already broken in our culture, and there is every reason to suppose that cloning would only make it harder to fix. Strangely, although Pence touches on worries raised about the family here and there, he offers no sustained discussion of the impact of cloning on family. Instead, he brands such concern "hypocritical" on the grounds that there are other, more immediate steps we could take to protect families and children without bothering about cloning.[27] This ad hominem plainly does not rebut, or even address, the charge that human cloning could greatly exacerbate an already dangerously unstable social situation.

I argue that conducting and applying (supposedly) scientific research is a pretty flimsy excuse for affronting human dignity.

Human cloning may thus deprive the clone of real parents. She may have many quasiparents, but one ground for worry is that none may be tied to her in the role of protector that a child's parents traditionally occupy. This danger is aggravated to the extent that the clone's parents may be more likely than those of other children to have produced her merely as a means to their own ends (e.g., providing tissue for donation to other children) and to treat her accordingly.

Cloning demeans the cloned

There are other grounds for legitimate concern about particular forms of human cloning, but I will not pursue them here. Rather, I want to make a few remarks about one of the more serious objections to human cloning as intrinsically and decisively wrong. That is the claim that it wrongs the person cloned by degrading him. It strikes me as so transparently demeaning to a human being to make him a product of technological manufacture that it is difficult to understand why some people claim not to see it. This is *not* the way we have ever treated human beings; it *is* the way we have always treated the subhuman things we regard as wholly subject to our will. Thus, in cloning a human person is treated in a way otherwise reserved only for subhuman beings. It is hard to know a better definition of degrading or depreciating. Consider a religious perspective. For half a millennium, Trinitarians have praised God the Son as equal to the Father precisely as "begotten, not made." The clone, however, is made, not begotten.[28] Even some advocates of cloning consider it replication, not reproduction. It is hard to see equal treatment, much less acknowledgment of human equality, when one person is planned and designed by another and then manufactured to the latter's specifications. Of course, some people twist IVF and even sexual procreation in these directions. That shows not that these new perversions are morally unproblematic, but that they should be avoided and condemned everywhere and that forms of reproduction that facilitate or encourage them have a heavy moral presumption against them.

There is little to show that cloning would do much to protect rights, alleviate injustice, avoid treachery, promote virtue, or thwart vice.

Nevertheless, Ruth Macklin told the NBAC, "If objectors to cloning can identify no greater harm than a supposed affront to the dignity of the human species, that is a flimsy basis on which to erect barriers to scientific research and its applications."[29] The report does not reproduce the context of her remarks, but it is important to observe that this quotation is not an argument but merely an assertion of her value ordering. I argue that conducting and applying (supposedly) scientific research is a pretty flimsy excuse for affronting human dignity. Of course, the person produced by cloning would not have existed but for this degradation. Some argue that this shows the act was not a net harm to her.[30] Even if that is correct, it does not suffice to show it is not a sufficient offense against her to render the act impermissible. After all, harm matters morally only insofar as it is a way of wronging someone. If harm is so narrowly defined that degrading someone is not harming her, then that only means that there are other ways of wronging people. So failure to harm does not entail failure to wrong. None of this means that the cloned person is subhuman, unequal, a thing to be used rather than a person to be respected. Rather, the argument presupposes just the opposite. That is why cloning is a degradation.[31]

In any case, pace Professor Macklin and others, scientific research is important, but we can do without it, as we did for most of our history. In contrast, it is doubtful that there is any secure foundation for human rights except in the inherent dignity of the individual. Thus, the Preamble to the 1948 *Universal Declaration of Human Rights* begins, "Whereas recognition of the inherent dignity and of the equal and inalienable rights of all members of the human family is the foundation of freedom, justice, and peace in the world." The first article, similarly, begins, "All human beings are born free and equal in dignity and rights."[32] The nature, source, limits, preconditions, and normative requirements of dignity could be made clearer, of course, as most important moral concepts could. That is a large part of the work of analytical moral philosophy. However, any suggestion that until this work is completed we should banish this concept—or the related concepts of rights, respect, and deference—from our discussion of the morality of human cloning should be regarded as we would the suggestion that we banish from bioethical discussions such controversial and imprecise concepts as cause, benefit, harm, or health until their conceptual clarification has been completed. We should greet it with derision.

If, as I maintain, all human cloning is wrong as a degradation of the one cloned, it may still be that some special forms of cloning are worse for special reasons. Thus, cloning *for* sex selection, to create tissue donors, to make "better babies," to replicate oneself, and so on, further demean the child to the extent that they value her simply for her use and characteristics rather than her nature. Cloning of human multiples is especially repugnant. Cloning from grandparents and other ancestors is odious for the harm such arrangements may do this culture's already unstable family relationships.[33] Likewise, research toward human cloning should be rejected as immoral insofar as it destroys human "preembryos," encourages degrading views of humans as mere means to organs, pursues the loathsome eugenic project of "improving humanity" by manufacturing Pence's "superior children," and so on.

This research is morally impermissible in part for the reason Paul Ramsey identified: It is performed without informed consent from those experimented upon.[34] Some want to dismiss Ramsey's objection on the grounds that it is absurd to demand consent from someone to the very procedures that may bring him into existence. Of course, that is right, as Ramsey presumably knew.[35] What is unclear is why anyone should think this proves that such consent is inessential. There is no contradiction in saying that consent is required for morally acceptable research and also that it cannot be secured in some proposed research. What follows from this is simply what Ramsey said: The proposed research is impermissible. A defender of cloning experiments may not like this conclusion but still must give some rebuttal to Ramsey's argument.

Some may think they can use the commonly accepted principle that "ought" implies "can" to rebut Ramsey. After all, if this principle is correct, and if informed consent to the experiment cannot be secured, then the experimenter cannot be accused of wrongdoing for failing to secure it. Again, this is correct, but it does not effectively rebut Ramsey. For Ramsey's claim is not that the experimenter ought to (and, if the principle is correct, therefore can) secure consent. Rather, it is that the experimenter ought not to perform the experiment without consent. And the experimenter surely can refrain from performing the experiment without consent. He or she can abandon the experiment.

The case for human cloning

I think the case for human cloning is rather weak. There is little to show that cloning would do much to protect rights, alleviate injustice, avoid treachery, promote virtue, or thwart vice. I suggest that one effort to vindicate the justice of human cloning fails rather badly. However, what matters is that even if it succeeded in demonstrating that position on the question of morally acceptable public policy, it could still be that human cloning itself is morally wrong—always, inherently, and indefeasibly. In short, the morality of public policy here, as elsewhere, underdetermines the central moral issue of whether the practice itself is morally permissible.

Some defend human cloning on the grounds that it could help prevent genetic disease.[36] Of course, this would be good. However, until we have some evidence of the likelihood that it really help and, moreover, help in ways that could not otherwise be realized (or not otherwise be realized without great sacrifice), this reason is, to borrow Macklin's term, "flimsy."[37]

The same holds for the defense of human cloning as an aid to those afflicted with infertility.[38] How likely is it to help? How much? In what ways? What are the prospects for alternative approaches? Moreover, we should remember that although infertility is a genuine health dysfunction, there are already *many* legally permitted, and some morally permissible, ways of compensating to a greater and lesser extent (e.g., adoption, social volunteering, and assisted reproductive techniques). Insofar as human cloning is proposed simply to assuage those unwilling or unable to find such alternatives reasonable accommodations, the case for it is still weaker. There is in general no compelling moral reason to make sure everyone gets what she or he wants. Sometimes the proper approach to dissatisfaction is to change one's desires, as the Stoics knew. It is a lesson our culture needs to relearn, not least in these matters.

What is presented as a noble parental effort . . . will sometimes result simply in parents refusing any child not up to their standards of beauty.

Eugenicist fans of human cloning think it will improve the race.[39] This is no reason at all, for the supposed improvement is moral retrogression, as its vicious rhetoric of "superior children" should make manifest. This merely displays an insulting and socially dangerous view of illness and human limits. Healthier adults are not superior to others. The same holds for babies. The main reason some do not regard talk of "better babies" as offensive is that some people, offensively, view babies as functional items to be evaluated according to how well they serve others' purposes, especially the purposes for which they were made. This instrumental view of people is deeply wrongheaded and ugly, yet it is the mentality that animates much of the push for human cloning. There is a related point. Sometimes talk of preventing disease is a smokescreen for eugenic improvements, as indicated, for example, by Pence's enthusiasm for "changing our [human] natures."[40] What is presented as a noble parental effort to avoid such illnesses as obesity will sometimes result simply in parents refusing any child not up to their standards of beauty.

Some also endorse cloning as a reproductive right.[41] I do not know what the U.S. Supreme Court is willing to affirm as constitutional rights these days. However, there is no good reason to see a *moral* right here. Although people plainly have some moral rights over their reproductive activities, talk of a right over how one reproduces is fanciful. Somebody might as well argue that a right to vote entails that Internet voting must be made available because some people would choose to vote that way.

Pence claims that homosexuals have been denied genetic connection to their children and endorses human cloning as a mode of redress.[42] Again, this is not serious for the same reason it would be unserious to demand such redress for celibates, avowed or adventitious [accidental].[43]

Justice does not require cloning

Theoretically, one of the most interesting arguments in support of the morality of human cloning is the appeal to John Rawls's theory of justice. Closely following Rawls, Pence reasons that in the original position, behind Rawls's "veil of ignorance," a rational contractor unaware of which generation she belonged to would choose for those in any generation to seek "the best genetic endowment" for their successors.[44] From this, he concludes that justice requires that society take steps to secure that optimal inheritance, including research and ultimately use of human cloning. Unfortunately, I think this argument is based on a misunderstanding of both Rawls's earlier and later understandings of his theory. Rawls's earlier version of his theory, in his book *A Theory of Justice,* makes it explicit that his theoretical apparatus is designed only to secure principles for ensuring that what he calls "the basic structure of society" meets criteria for "social justice." So understood, the apparatus of the original position is misapplied when used to derive conclusions about whether various practices are morally licit. Even if one accepts Rawls's theory as he first proposed it, the most that the defender of human cloning could show with it is that society should not interfere with human cloning, not that cloning itself is morally permissible. Of course, I doubt that Rawls's early theory, if itself correct, really shows even that. That the goal of eliminating genetic disease is justified does not suffice to show that such means as cloning are themselves permissible. Indeed, the deontological element in Rawls makes it more difficult to derive such conclusion about means from premises simply about ends.

The theory from Rawls's later book, *Political Liberalism,* is still more narrowly circumscribed as a theory simply of political justice for reaching collective political decisions in societies with certain kinds of history, commitments, projects, self-conceptions, and so on. Again, it contains no conclusions about the permissibility of such nonpolitical practices as human cloning.

Human cloning . . . presents us with a different face of what has rightly been called the "anti-life culture" that infects our medicine.

On the whole, then, the case for human cloning as found in such works as Pence's is hardly compelling. For the most part, it does not deal in the graver moral realms of freeing people from injustice, ending vicious conduct, or attaining a deeper appreciation of what is valuable. Nor is it at all established that human cloning is likely to free real people from what any reasonable, objective observer would see as serious health deficits in someone's functioning as a human being. Rather, often the case largely reduces to the claim that human cloning may make some things go somewhat better for some people, largely by making things go more to their liking. In light, among other things, of the affront to human dignity and equality that human cloning appears to constitute, a much stronger kind of defense is needed to vindicate it morally.

In the end, human cloning merely presents us with a different face of what has rightly been called the "anti-life culture" that infects our medicine. It is another way of attacking human life, this time by degrading it rather than destroying it, by treating human life as something for us to bestow, and therefore of subordinate and only instrumental value. That other practices manifesting this mentality have won wide public acceptance in the last few decades does nothing to justify them, let alone human cloning.

Notes

I am grateful to the audience at University of San Francisco's 1998 conference "Human Cloning: Science, Ethics, and Public Policy" and to Victoria Wiesner and W. David Solomon for bibliographic materials.

1. Gina Kolata, "On Cloning Humans, 'Never' Turns into 'Why Not,'" *New York Times*, Dec. 2, 1997, p. A1. See also George Johnson, "Ethical Fears Aside, Science Plunges On," *New York Times*, Dec. 7, 1997, p. 6.

2. A usage note: Throughout, I talk simply of "human cloning." This is not as clear as it could be because the term can be applied to many different things. On this, see Gregory Pence, *Who's Afraid of Human Cloning?* (Lanham, Md.: Rowman & Littlefield, 1998), 11. However, many of these differences make little moral difference and it is important to resist the urge to drift into technical obscurity and lose the resonance of the more familiar term. Pence and others now prefer the term *nuclear somatic transfer* (ibid., 49). I demur, concerned lest this move, like the insistence on the term *preembryo* and similar moves, form part of a strategy of obfuscation and euphemism. On the strategy, with special reference to the terms *preembryo* and *nuclear somatic transfer* see Kolata, "On Cloning Humans," p. F4.

3. Pence, *Who's Afraid of Human Cloning?*, 123–25, 139, 165, and passim.

4. Ibid., 7.

5. Ibid., 65.

6. Ibid., 66.

7. Ibid., 70.

8. See Ronald Dworkin, "Assisted Suicide: What the Court Really Said," *New York Review of Books*, Sept. 25,1997, pp. 40–44. On Holland's troubles, see Herbert Hendin, *Seduced by Death: Doctors, Patients, and the Dutch Cure* (New York: W.W. Norton, 1996).

9. Pence, *Who's Afraid of Human Cloning?*, 130.

10. Richard Lewontin, "Confusion over Cloning," *New York Review of Books*, Oct. 23,1997, p. 23.

11. Pence, *Who's Afraid of Human Cloning?*, 35,153.

12. Ibid., 80.

13. Ibid., 97.

14. Ibid., 81.

15. Ibid., 5, 6.

16. Peter Singer, "Sidgwick and Reflective Equilibrium," *Monist* 58 (1974): 516, quoted in Pence, *Who's Afraid of Human Cloning?*, 64.

17. Note, too, that whatever Mill may have thought, it is no longer plausible to maintain that utilitarianism can stand without support from our intuitions either in its consequentialist account of what actions are right, its aggregative and sum ranking account of what distributional schemes or states of affairs are better, or its account of the maximand. Indeed, the very decision to interpret its central principle as that of maximizing what is good rather than one of minimizing what is bad is itself usually decided on the basis of intuition. There is no obvious warrant for Singer's—and, by implication, Pence's—confidence that all these intuitions will be trustworthy and pristine whereas intuitions about the immorality of such practices as cloning are corrupted. For an introduction to some of the issues over utilitarians' competing understandings of happiness as pleasure or preference satisfaction, negative utilitarianism, act utilitarianism versus rule and other forms of indirect utilitarianism, whether the happiness principle should be used by agents in practical deliberation or only by critics in retrospective assessment, and other related issues, see Geoffrey Scarre, *Utilitarianism* (London: Routledge, 1996).

18. See, for example, John A. Robertson, "The Question of Human Cloning," *Hastings Center Report*, Mar./Apr. 1994, p. 11. See also Richard McCormick's response, "Blastomere Separation: Some Concerns," ibid., 14–16.

19. Pence, Who's *Afraid of Human Cloning?*, 142.

20. As an interpretation of Mill, the problem is that it is not consistent with the utility principle to maintain that there are actions immune from moral assessment.

21. Pence, *Who's Afraid of Human Cloning?*, 145.

22. It is not fully clear that this makes it sexist because, although the gestating mother must be a woman, of course, even males involved in desexed reproduction and child-rearing will similarly be demeaned by their participation.

23. Pence, *Who's Afraid of Human Cloning?*, 79.

24. Or still worse, I suppose, a postmodernist one. As an example, see Michel Foucault's three-volume history of sexuality, *A History of Sexuality* (New York: Vintage, 1990).

25. I ignore the complication of mitochondrial genes.

26. Lewontin, "Confusion over Cloning," 21; Pence, *Who's Afraid of Human Cloning?*, 122–23.

27. Pence, *Who's Afraid of Human Cloning?*, 139–40.

28. See Albert S. Moraczewski, "Cloning Testimony," *Ethics and Medics* 22 (May 1997): 3; Pontifical Academy for Life, "Human Cloning Is Immoral," *The Pope Speaks* 43 (Jan./Feb. 1998): 27–32.

29. National Bioethics Advisory Commission, *Cloning Human Beings* (Rockville, Md.: NBAC, 1997), 71.

30. See the discussion in ibid., 65–66.

31. Moraczewski, "Cloning Testimony," 3.

32. See, for example, the text reproduced in the periodical *First Things* 82 (Apr. 1998): 28–30. For a discussion, especially on the importance and

ground of human dignity, see the Ramsey Colloquium, "On Human Rights," ibid., 18–22. See also Richard Doerflinger, *National Conference of Catholic Bishops' Statement at U.S. Capitol* (Washington, D.C.: NCCB, Jan. 29, 1998); Moraczewski, "Cloning Testimony"; and Pontifical Academy for Life, "Human Cloning Is Immoral."

33. It may be that cloning *for* male or female homosexuals, cloning the superannuated, and so on are also to be condemned for similar reasons.

34. See Paul Ramsey, *Fabricated Man* (New Haven, Conn.: Yale University Press, 1970). See also Pence, *Who's Afraid of Human Cloning?*, 52.

35. Notice, however, that it begs an important question about the moral status of the embryo (and "preembryo") to assume that there is no person at all involved in cases of experimentation on a human embryo. I am grateful to Al Howsepian for focussing my attention on this element in the dispute between Ramsey and Pence. The common ground in such cases is that there is no person in a position to give or withhold consent.

36. Pence, *Who's Afraid of Human Cloning?*, 101–106.

37. At least here it can be said that human cloning would pursue this end in a less morally outrageous way, that is, by genetically healing those with genetic disease markers, as compared with IVF, where the effort is not to help any real person but to prevent conception of the diseased or to destroy those marked before they can be born.

38. Pence, *Who's Afraid of Human Cloning?*, 106ff.

39. Ibid., 166–70.

40. "A frequent corollary to the fatalist viewpoint is that human nature is not to be trusted with any new knowledge. Any attempt to change our natures [in this view] will produce dark consequences" (ibid., 124; see also 165). Note that Pence here talks as if gaining new knowledge and trying to change human nature were the same thing.

41. Ibid., 44, 45,101.

42. Ibid., 114.

43. Moreover, it merely encourages irresponsibility to disconnect natural effects from causes in this way. In light of what we said about the family, it can be seen that bioengineering is partner of dangerous, unproven social experiments. Those who, like Pence, pride themselves on the empiricism of their approach need to attend more closely to the safety issues surrounding these social experiments.

44. Pence, *Who's Afraid of Human Cloning?*, 112–14.

Organizations to Contact

The editors have compiled the following list of organizations and websites concerned with the issues debated in this book. The descriptions are derived from materials provided by the organizations themselves. All have publications or information available for interested readers. The list was compiled on the date of publication of the present volume; the information provided here may change. Be aware that many organizations take several weeks or longer to respond to inquiries, so allow as much time as possible.

American Crop Protection Association
1156 Fifteenth St. NW, Suite 400, Washington, DC 20005
(202) 296-1585 • fax: (202) 463-0474
e-mail: member_services@acpa.org • website: www.acpa.org

The ACPA promotes the environmentally sound use of crop protection products, including bioengineered plants containing Bt and other pesticide genes, for the economical production of safe, high-quality, abundant food and other crops. It represents the pesticide industry. Its website includes general information about plant biotechnology and papers and news releases describing the benefits and safety of genetically engineered crops, such as "New Research Suggests Bt-Corn Not Harmful to Monarch Butterfly."

American Society of Law, Medicine, and Ethics
765 Commonwealth Ave., Suite 1634, Boston, MA 02215
(617) 262-4990 • fax: (617) 437-7596
e-mail: info@aslme.org • website: www.aslme.org

This group acts as a forum for discussion of issues including the ethics of genetic engineering. Its material is aimed primarily at professionals in the fields of health care and law. It publishes two quarterly journals, *Journal of Law, Medicine, and Ethics* and *American Journal of Law and Medicine*. Its website includes a number of papers on deciphering and engineering the human genome, such as "Parental Autonomy and the Obligation Not to Harm One's Child Genetically."

Biotechnology Industry Organization (BIO)
1625 K St. NW, Suite 1100, Washington, DC 20006
(202) 857-0244
website: www.bio.org

The Biotechnology Industry Organization represents biotechnology companies, academic institutions, state biotechnology centers, and related organizations that support the use of biotechnology in agriculture, health care, and other fields. BIO works to educate the public about biotechnology and responds to concerns about the safety and ethics of genetic engineering and related technologies. Its website includes an introductory guide to biotechnology as well as links to other biotechnology websites and press releases and position papers on bioethics, food and agriculture, and similar topics.

Center for Bioethics and Human Dignity (CBHD)
2065 Half Day Rd., Bannockburn, IL 60015
(847) 317-8180 • fax: (847) 317-8153
e-mail: cbhd@cbhd.org • website: www.bioethix.org

CBHD is an international education center whose purpose is to bring Christian perspectives to bear on contemporary bioethical challenges facing society. It opposes the alteration of human genes. It publishes the newsletter *Dignity* as well as booklets, videos, and other materials. Its website contains articles (for example, "Genetic Intervention: The Ethical Challenges Ahead") and public statements, issue overviews, bibliographies, links, and publications for sale.

Center for Food Safety and Applied Nutrition
200 C St. SW, Washington, DC 20204
(888) 463-6332
website: http://vm.cfsan.fda.gov/list.html

The Center for Food Safety and Applied Nutrition is the part of the federal government's Food and Drug Administration (FDA) that regulates genetically engineered food crops. The center's website includes a collection of papers on biotechnology and the FDA's regulation of the biotechnology industry, including "Draft Guidance for Industry: Voluntary Labeling Indicating Whether Foods Have or Have Not Been Developed Using Bioengineering," posted January 2001.

Council for Responsible Genetics (CRG)
5 Upland Rd., Suite 3, Cambridge, MA 02140
(617) 868-0870 • fax: (617) 491-5344
e-mail: crg@gene-watch.org • website: www.gene-watch.org

The Council for Responsible Genetics is a national nonprofit organization of scientists and others devoted to encouraging public debate about the social, ethical, and environmental implications of new genetic technologies. It works to provide members of the public with clear and understandable information on genetic innovations so that they can participate in decision making about genetic technology and its implementation. Material on CRG's website includes a petition titled "No Patents on Life," a position paper on manipulation of the human germline, and news alerts.

Foundation on Economic Trends (FET)
1660 L St. NW, Suite 216, Washington, DC 20036
(202) 466-2823 • fax: (202) 429-9602
e-mail: office@biotechcentury.org • website: www.biotechcentury.org

Founded by science critic and author Jeremy Rifkin, the foundation is a non-profit organization whose mission is to examine emerging trends in science and technology and their impacts on the environment, the economy, culture, and society. FET works to educate the public about topics such as gene patenting, commercial eugenics, genetic discrimination, and genetically altered food. It has proposed a moratorium on somatic (individual) gene therapy using viruses to transmit genes into human cells and favors labeling of genetically altered food. Information on these positions is available on the organization's website.

Future Generations
e-mail: vancourt@eugenics.net
website: www.eugenics.net

This group, headed by Marian Van Court, strives to leave a legacy of good health, high intelligence, and noble character to future generations by humanitarian eugenics, or judicious altering of the human genome. The organization's website includes a number of articles explaining and defending its point of view.

The Hastings Center
Route 9D, Garrison, NY 10524-5555
(914) 424-4040 • fax: (914) 424-4545
website: www.thehastingscenter.org

The Hastings Center is an independent research institute that explores fundamental ethical issues in health, medicine, and the environment, including modification of human genes. It publishes a bimonthly journal, the *Hastings Center Report*, and other papers, some of which can be viewed on its website.

Human Cloning Foundation
PMB 143, 1100 Hammond Dr., Suite 410A, Atlanta, GA 30328
e-mail: RWicker@gateway.net • website: www.humancloning.org

The foundation is a nonprofit organization that promotes education about human cloning and gene alteration and emphasizes the positive aspects of these technologies. Its website contains numerous articles and fact sheets supporting human cloning.

Human Genome Diversity Project (HGDP)
c/o Morrison Institute for Population and Resource Studies
371 Sierra Mall (Gilbert 116), MC 5020, Stanford University
Stanford, CA 94305-5020
(650) 723-7518 • fax: (650) 725-8244
e-mail: morrinst@stanford.edu
website: www.stanford.edu/group/morrinst/hgdp.html

The Human Genome Diversity Project is an international project that seeks to understand the diversity and unity of the human species by collecting DNA samples from a variety of indigenous groups. The project is currently in its planning stages. Several documents are available on its website, including the model ethical protocol (procedure) for collecting DNA samples and answers to frequently asked questions about the HGDP.

Institute for Food and Development Policy (Food First)
398 60th St., Oakland, CA 94608
(510) 654-4400 • fax: (510) 654-4551
e-mail: foodfirst@foodfirst.org • website: www.foodfirst.org

The Institute for Food and Development Policy, better known as Food First, is a member-supported, nonprofit think tank and education-for-action center working to highlight root causes and value-based solutions to hunger and poverty around the world. It produces books, reports, articles, films, workshops, and other educational material and action plans for the public, policymakers, activists, students, and the media. Papers available on its website include "Ten Reasons Why Biotechnology Will Not Ensure Food Security" and "Critiquing Biotechnology and Industrial Agriculture."

International Food Information Council Foundation
1100 Connecticut Ave. NW, Suite 430, Washington, DC 20036
e-mail: foodinfo@ific.health.org • website: http://ificinfo.health.org

IFIC aims to bridge the gap between science and communications by collecting and distributing scientific information on food safety, nutrition, and health to opinion leaders and consumers. Its website includes newsbriefs such as "More U.S. Consumers See Potential Benefits to Food Biotechnology." Single copies of publications, such as "Food Biotechnology Resource Kit," may be ordered free online.

International Food Policy Research Institute (IFPRI)
2033 K St. NW, Washington, DC 20006
(202) 862-5600 • fax: (202) 467-4439
e-mail: ifpri@cgiar.org • website: www.ifpri.cgiar.org

IFPRI is the U.S. center of the Consultative Group on International Agricultural Research (CGIAR). Its mission is to identify and analyze policies for sustainably meeting the food needs of the developing world. It publishes a quarterly newsletter, *IFPRI Perspectives,* and booklets such as "World Food Prospects," some of which can be ordered free online.

National Bioethics Advisory Commission (NBAC)
6705 Rockledge Dr., Suite 700, Rockville, MD 20892-7979
(301) 402-4242 • fax: (301) 480-6900
website: www.bioethics.gov

NBAC is a federal agency that sets guidelines governing the ethical conduct of research. It works to protect the rights and welfare of human research subjects and governs the management and use of genetic information. Its published reports include *Cloning Human Beings* and *Ethical Issues in Human Stem Cell Research.*

National Human Genome Research Institute (NHGRI)
9000 Rockville Pike, Bethesda, MD 20892
(301) 402-0911 • fax: (301) 402-0837
website: www.nhgri.nih.gov

Sponsored by the National Institutes of Health, the federal government's primary agency for the support of biomedical research, NHGRI heads the Human Genome Project, the federally funded effort to map all human genes. Information about the Human Genome Project, including its ethical, legal, and social implications, is available at NHGRI's website.

Rural Advancement Foundation International (RAFI)
110 Osborne St., Suite 202, Winnipeg MB R3L 1Y5 Canada
(204) 453-5259 • fax: (204) 925-8034
e-mail: rafi@rafi.org • website: www.rafi.org

RAFI is an international, nongovernmental organization dedicated to the conservation and sustainable improvement of agricultural biodiversity and to the socially responsible development of technologies useful to rural societies. It opposes agricultural biotechnology, especially as managed by large companies, and patenting of genetic material. It publishes a communique four to six times a year as well as occasional papers and other publications, many of which are available online. An example is "In Search of Higher Ground: The Intellectual Property Challenge to Public Agricultural Research and Human Rights."

U.S. Department of Agriculture (USDA)
Animal and Plant Health Inspection Service (APHIS)
14th and Independence Ave. SW, Washington, DC 20250
e-mail: john.t.turner@usda.gov • website: www.aphis.usda.gov/biotechnology

The USDA is one of three federal agencies, along with the Environmental Protection Agency (EPA) and the Food and Drug Administration (FDA), primarily responsible for regulating biotechnology in the United States. The USDA's Animal and Plant Health Inspection Service (APHIS) conducts research on the safety of genetically engineered organisms, helps form government policy on agricultural biotechnology, and provides information to the public about these technologies. The APHIS website includes policy statements on biotechnology, a description of the role of the USDA and its agencies in regulating agricultural biotechnology, and research reports, including "Impacts of Adopting Genetically Engineered Crops in the United States."

Additional Internet Resources

The following websites contain a wealth of information for students and others interested in learning more about genetic engineering and ethical issues involving this technology.

Access Excellence
website: www.accessexcellence.org

This site is aimed at teachers and students and contains news about biotechnology, a history of biotechnology (the Biotech Chronicles), educational activities, and links to many other sites related to biotechnology and genetics.

Bioethicsline
website: http://igm.nlm.nih.gov

Sponsored by the National Library of Medicine, part of the National Institutes of Health, Bioethicsline is an online medical database. It offers annotated bibliographies on the ethics of technologies such as gene therapy and human cloning.

National Biotechnology Information Facility (NBIF)
website: http://nbif.org

This website contains a variety of games, activities, and other materials that educate students about biotechnology and an Internet Resources section that includes more than 3,300 annotated links to biotechnology-related sites.

Bibliography

Books

William R. Clark — *The New Healers*. New York: Oxford University Press, 1997.

Eric S. Grace — *Biotech Unzipped: Promises and Realities*. Washington, DC: Joseph Henry Press, 1997.

Ruth Hubbard and Elijah Wald — *Exploding the Gene Myth*. Boston: Beacon Press, 1997.

Leon R. Kass and James Q. Wilson — *The Ethics of Human Cloning*. Washington, DC: AEI Press, 1998.

Glenn McGee — *The Perfect Baby: A Pragmatic Approach to Genetics*. Lanham, MD: Rowman & Littlefield, 1997.

M.L. Rantala and Arthur J. Milgram, eds. — *Cloning: For and Against*. Chicago: Open Court, 1999.

Jeremy Rifkin — *The Biotech Century*. New York: Jeremy P. Tarcher, 1998.

Thomas A. Shannon — *Genetic Engineering: A Documentary History*. Westport, CT: Greenwood Publishing Group, 1999.

Thomas A. Shannon — *Made in Whose Image: Genetic Engineering and Christian Ethics*. Amherst, NY: Humanity Books, 1999.

Lee M. Silver — *Remaking Eden: How Genetic Engineering and Cloning Will Transform the American Family*. New York: Avon, 1998.

Martin Teitel and Kimberly A. Wilson — *Genetically Engineered Food: Changing the Nature of Nature*. Rochester, VT: Park Street Press, 1999.

James D. Torr, ed. — *Opposing Viewpoints: Genetic Engineering*. San Diego, CA: Greenhaven Press, 2001.

Jon Turney — *Frankenstein's Footsteps: Science, Genetics and Popular Culture*. New Haven, CT: Yale University Press, 1998.

Lisa Yount — *Contemporary Issues Companion: Cloning*. San Diego, CA: Greenhaven Press, 2000.

Lisa Yount — *Library in a Book: Biotechnology and Genetic Engineering*. New York: Facts On File, 2000.

Periodicals

Ronald Bailey — "The Twin Paradox," *Reason*, May 1997. Available from the Reason Foundation, 3415 S. Sepulveda Blvd., Suite 400, Los Angeles, CA 90034.

Paul R. Billings, Ruth Hubbard, and Stuart A. Newman — "Human Germline Gene Modification: A Dissent," *Lancet*, May 29, 1999.

Kathryn S. Brown	"Food with Attitude," *Discover*, March 2000.
Business Week	"Are Bio-Foods Safe?" December 20, 1999.
Lisa Sowle Cahill	"Human Primordial Stem Cells: The New Biotech World Order," *The Hastings Center Report*, March 1999. Available from The Hastings Center, Route 9D, Garrison, NY 10524-5555.
Thomas W. Clark	"Playing God, Carefully," *The Humanist*, May 2000.
Kevin Clarke	"Unnatural Selection," *U.S. Catholic*, January 2000. Available from *U.S. Catholic*, 205 W. Monroe St., Chicago, IL 60606.
Ronnie Cummins	"Problems with Genetic Engineering," *Synthesis/Regeneration*, Winter 1999. Available from Gateway Green Alliance/Green Party of St. Louis, P.O. Box 8094, St. Louis, MO 63156.
David Ehrenfeld	"A Techno-Pox upon the Land," *Harper's Magazine*, October 1997.
Futurist	"Biotechnology and Future Food Supply," July 2000. Available from the World Future Society, 7910 Woodmont Ave., Suite 450, Bethesda, MD 20814.
Thomas Hayden	"Monkeying with Nature," *U.S. News & World Report*, January 22, 2001.
Mae-Wan Ho	"The Unholy Alliance," *The Ecologist*, July-August 1997.
Marguerite Lamb et al.	"Brave New Food," *Mother Earth News*, April 2000. Available from *Mother Earth News*, P.O. Box 56302, Boulder, CO 80322-6302.
Klaus M. Leisinger	"Yes: Stop Blocking Progress," *Foreign Policy*, Summer 2000. Available from Carnegie Endowment for International Peace, 1779 Massachusetts Ave., NW, Washington, DC 20036-2103.
Mary Midgley	"Biotechnology and Monstrosity: Why We Should Pay Attention to the 'Yuk Factor,'" *The Hastings Center Report*, September 2000.
National Catholic Reporter	"Designer Babies, Anyone?" October 22, 1999. Available from *National Catholic Reporter*, 115 E. Armour Blvd., Kansas City, MO 64111.
Virginia I. Postrel	"Fatalist Attraction: The Dubious Case Against Fooling Mother Nature," *Reason*, July 1997.
C.S. Prakash	"Hungry for Biotech," *Technology Review*, July 2000.
Susan Reed	"My Sister, My Clone," *Time*, February 19, 2001.
Jeremy Rifkin	"Future Pharming," *Animals*, May-June 1998. Available from the Massachusetts Society for the Prevention of Cruelty to Animals, 350 S. Huntington Ave., Boston, MA 02130.

Jeremy Rifkin	"The Ultimate Therapy," *Tikkun*, May-June 1998. Available from *Tikkun*, 2107 Van Ness Ave., Suite 302, San Francisco, CA 94109.
Peter Rosset	"The Parable of the Golden Snail," *The Nation*, December 27, 1999.
Ismael Sarageldin	"Biotechnology and Food Security in the 21st Century," *Science*, July 16, 1999.
Pamela Schaeffer	"Revolution in Biology Drives Revolution in Theology, Ethics and Law," *National Catholic Reporter*, October 22, 1999.
Ricarda Steinbrecher	"What Is Wrong with Nature?" *Synthesis/Regeneration*, Winter 1999.
Mark Strauss	"When Malthus Meets Mendel," *Foreign Policy*, Summer 2000.
Laura Tangley	"Engineering the Harvest," *U.S. News & World Report*, March 13, 2000.
Laura Tangley	"Of Genes, Grain, and Grocers," *U.S. News & World Report*, April 10, 2000.
Larry Thompson	"Are Bioengineered Foods Safe?" *FDA Consumer*, January 2000.
Time	"Grains of Hope," July 31, 2000.
Colin Tudge	"When It's Right to Be a Luddite," *New Statesman*, April 24, 2000.
Roger Wrubel	"Biotechnology: Right or Wrong?" *Bioscience*, March 1998.

Index